THE PUBLISHER GRATEFULLY ACKNOWLEDGES THE GENEROUS SUPPORT OF THE ROBERT AND MERYL SELIG ENDOWMENT FUND IN FILM STUDIES, IN MEMORY OF ROBERT W. SELIG, OF THE UNIVERSITY OF CALIFORNIA PRESS FOUNDATION.

BACKSTORY 5

ALSO BY PATRICK McGILLIGAN

AS AUTHOR

Cagney: The Actor as Auteur
Robert Altman: Jumping off the Cliff
George Cukor: A Double Life
Jack's Life: A Biography of Jack Nicholson
Fritz Lang: The Nature of the Beast
Film Crazy: Interviews with Hollywood Legends
Clint, the Life and Legend: A Biography of Clint Eastwood
Alfred Hitchcock: A Life in Darkness and Light
Oscar Micheaux: The Great and Only

AS EDITOR

Backstory: Interviews with Screenwriters of Hollywood's Golden Age
Backstory 2: Interviews with Screenwriters of the 1940s and 1950s
Backstory 3: Interviews with Screenwriters of the 1960s
Backstory 4: Interviews with Screenwriters of the 1970s and 1980s
Six by Robert Riskin
Tender Comrades: A Backstory of the Blacklist (with Paul Buhle)

BACKSTORY 5

INTERVIEWS WITH SCREENWRITERS OF THE 1990s

EDITED AND WITH AN INTRODUCTION BY

PATRICK McGILLIGAN

UNIVERSITY OF CALIFORNIA PRESS   BERKELEY LOS ANGELES LONDON

University of California Press, one of the most distinguished university presses in the United States, enriches lives around the world by advancing scholarship in the humanities, social sciences, and natural sciences. Its activities are supported by the UC Press Foundation and by philanthropic contributions from individuals and institutions. For more information, visit www.ucpress.edu.

University of California Press
Berkeley and Los Angeles, California

University of California Press, Ltd.
London, England

Library of Congress Cataloging-in-Publication Data

Backstory 5 : interviews with screenwriters of the 1990s / edited and with an introduction by Patrick McGilligan.

p. cm.

Includes bibliographical references and index.

ISBN 978-0-520-25105-2 (cloth : alk. paper)

ISBN 978-0-520-26039-9 (pbk. : alk. paper)

1. Screenwriters—California—Los Angeles—Interviews. I. McGilligan, Patrick.

PN1998.2.B3452 2010

812'.5409—dc22 2009028718

Manufactured in the United States of America

19 18 17 16 15 14 13 12 11 10

10 9 8 7 6 5 4 3 2 1

This book is printed on Natures Book, which contains 50% post-consumer waste and meets the minimum requirements of ANSI/NISO Z39.48-1992 (R 1997) (*Permanence of Paper*).

FOR JOEL,
FAITHFUL READER AND FRIEND

CONTENTS

ACKNOWLEDGMENTS

The Albert Brooks, Jean-Claude Carrière, Richard LaGravenese, John Sayles, Tom Stoppard, and Rudy Wurlitzer interviews are used with the permission of their authors. The individual authors retain their copyrights for any uses of their interviews beyond any versions or editions of *Backstory 5*.

The Albert Brooks interview was previously published in *Film Comment*, July–August 1999. The John Hughes interview was originally published in *Lollipop*, issue no. 47, Spring 1999. A version of the David Koepp interview was presented in June 2008 as an online exclusive of *Writer's Digest*. Portions of the Richard LaGravenese interview first appeared in the September–October 2007 issue of *Creative Screenwriting*. Portions of the Barry Levinson interview were published in *The Writer*, May 2008.

PATRICK McGILLIGAN

INTRODUCTION

The world keeps turning, spinning madly one might say, and here we are at the fifth volume of the *Backstory* series, more than two decades after the publication of my first book of interviews with Hollywood screenwriters of the golden age.

Much has changed since the first book; in particular, there is now a common understanding and widespread use of the word *backstory*. I had to ask around about it in the early 1980s. The *New York Times* columnist William Safire, writing about its proliferation, credited the initial *Backstory* with helping to bring the old word into vogue again.[1] Bless him. "Unfortunately for etymologists," Safire wrote, "no interviewer asked the early screenwriters if they ever used the word *backstory*." But I did, and they said they used the word to mean the "backstory" of the characters and plot of a script; that's where the title of the first book, *Backstory: Interviews with Screenwriters of Hollywood's Golden Age*, came from.

I have used it more broadly to signify the backstory of the profession, as well as the backstory of a particular writer, specific script, or film. The series up to now has tried to tell the backstory or history of the screenwriting craft, dating roughly from the late silent era up through the 1980s, which is the rubric of *Backstory 4*. I recommend the earlier volumes to you, if the word or series is new to you.

Hollywood keeps evolving, and so does screenwriting. Pen and pencil are for diehards now, as are three-by-five cards for plotting. Typewriters are out, computers in. Living in Los Angeles is also out; only three of the distinguished interviewees in *Backstory 5* actually live in the Hollywood vicinity. Nowadays some top names prefer to live on the East Coast, flying—and whizzing their e-mails—back and forth from coast to coast. The business is still centered on Hollywood production, but the ownership of the studios constantly revolves, and the market is more than ever global.

One thing remains fixed, stable, still true. The script is where the film starts, the origin of ideas and the foundation of excellence. This has been the credo of the *Backstory* series—an "anti-director-as-auteur" credo, if you will: the script is the key element defining quality filmmaking.

The interview subjects profiled in *Backstory 5: Interviews with Screenwriters of the 1990s* include some of the best known, highest paid, most garlanded, most dependable writers of the decade. As usual, I have fudged the frame of the book—"the 1990s"—to include favorite writers (regardless of the decade in which he or she peaked) and to reflect a range of styles and approaches.

Funnyman **ALBERT BROOKS** is always a welcome presence as an actor in films, but as writer-director he is justly acclaimed for a series of personal, sometimes semiautobiographical comedies exploring dysfunctional America, including *The Muse,* from 1999, which mocks Hollywood from the point of view of a beleaguered screenwriter.

JEAN-CLAUDE CARRIÈRE will always be linked with Luis Buñuel for the exceptional films they made together in the 1960s and 1970s, but Carrière has amassed more than one hundred credits over his long career. These encompass important films for leading filmmakers of several countries besides his native France, including the United States.

A child of Hollywood who first became a household name as a journalist, **NORA EPHRON** has carved out a unique niche in writing-directing, which is still predominantly a boys' club, with award-winning smash-hit romantic comedies that blend her wry feminism with traditional Hollywood formulas.

Playwright and author **RONALD HARWOOD** has a sideline of writing serious, intelligent films that dates back to the early 1960s. I'd say his career was capped by an Oscar for the screenplay of *The Pianist* in 2002, but he shows no signs of slowing down, with an Oscar nomination in 2007 for adapting *The Diving Bell and the Butterfly* and with more scripts still in the works.

The elusive **JOHN HUGHES** is the undisputed champion of "teen" movies as well as the creator of several box-office triumphs that fall outside the teen category. His heyday as writer-director-producer was in the 1980s and early 1990s. Although he no longer directs, he remains prolific, often under pseudonyms.

DAVID KOEPP writes often for Steven Spielberg and Brian DePalma and has participated in the *Jurassic Park, Mission: Impossible, Spider-Man,* and *Indiana Jones* blockbuster franchises. But he also steps outside the mold to write (and sometimes direct) his own taut originals "on spec"—independently and without advance payment.

RICHARD LaGRAVENESE, an entrenched homegrown New Yorker, made a splash with the Oscar-nominated *The Fisher King* in 1991 and has never looked back, writing major movies for Clint Eastwood, Diane Keaton, Barbara Streisand, and Robert Redford. Like Koepp and many other A-list writers, in recent years LaGravenese has successfully turned to directing his own scripts.

BARRY LEVINSON started out with television variety shows and wacky Mel Brooks comedies before vaulting to the top of the "hyphenate" ranks of writer-directors with his autobiographical *Diner* in 1982. The "Baltimore films" made him one of Hollywood's most admired writers, but he also directs films he does not write, including *Rain Man* from 1988, for which he won an Oscar for Best Director.

If there is a seminal film of the 1990s, it is *Forrest Gump,* for which **ERIC ROTH** won an Oscar for Best Adapted Screenplay, one of four nominations in a quietly auspicious career dating back four decades. A pure writer with no wish to direct, Roth closely collaborates (sometimes without credit) with Hollywood's top-drawer filmmakers.

JOHN SAYLES is an exemplar of the independent, iconoclastic screenwriter, a writer first and foremost (before being a director, producer, or actor) who has been making politically outspoken films on his own terms for twenty-five years, while continuing to hire himself out as a script doctor on mainstream Hollywood films.

One of England's greatest playwrights, **TOM STOPPARD** is another writer who has dabbled in projects with Steven Spielberg, as well as with Joseph Losey, Rainer Werner Fassbinder, and Terry Gilliam; though, when such script work includes a 1994 Oscar for *Shakespeare in Love,* it really ought not be called dabbling.

BARBARA TURNER is a free spirit who has flown under the radar for forty years. Once an actress in Robert Altman's circle, Turner wrote *Petulia,* her first major script, in 1966, thrived as a television writer for two decades, then returned to big-screen credits with *Georgia* (1995)—a starring vehicle for her own daughter, Jennifer Jason-Leigh—the impressive *Pollock* (2000) for actor-director Ed Harris; and an autumnal film for Altman (*The Company,* 2003).

Cult figure **RUDY WURLITZER** has divided his career between literary and cinematic endeavors, collaborating (happily in some instances, less so in others) on quixotic films with the likes of Jim McBride, Monte Hellman, Sam Peckinpah, Robert Frank, Alex Cox, Carroll Ballard, Michelangelo Antonioni, and Bernardo Bertolucci.

The youngest of the bunch is Koepp, who was born in 1963, around the time Carrière, Turner, and Harwood were embarking on their maiden film scripts. The intention of each volume of *Backstory* is to present a representative group portrait of screenwriters of a certain epoch, but in this case, it is more than ever a snapshot of a profession in motion. Whatever might be said about the empty commercialism of contemporary Hollywood, even as they were being interviewed, each of these reliably astute, fierce-minded writers—including the most veteran among them—was busy, busy, busy. They had to schedule Q-and-A sessions between phone calls with important directors, answer final e-mail queries amid trips to sets or editing rooms, and beg off additional questions to return to work on promising film projects in progress.

NOTE

1 William Safire, "On Language," *New York Times Sunday Magazine*, August 7, 2005.

INTERVIEW BY **GAVIN SMITH**

ALBERT BROOKS ME GENERATION EVERYMAN

In Albert Brooks's comedy *The Muse* (1999), a Hollywood screenwriter (played by Brooks) attempts to reignite his stalled career by employing the services of a muse (Sharon Stone). Descended from one of the nine Muses of Greek myth, she boasts an impressive track record of divinely inspired careers—at one point she and Brooks bump into Rob Reiner, who exclaims, "Thank you for *The American President.*" Expensive, demanding, and capricious, the muse rapidly takes over the screenwriter's life, requiring lavish treatment and eventually moving in with Brooks and his wife (Andie MacDowell).

Co-written by Brooks and Monica Johnson, this satire of Hollywood is embellished with sharp, frequently hilarious observation of its ritual humiliations and shallow social and professional interactions, with notable contributions from Jeff Bridges as a self-absorbed Oscar-winning screenwriter friend, Steven Wright as Stan Spielberg ("I'm Steven's cousin"), and Martin Scorsese in a self-parodying cameo. But at its core is the spectacle of a rational, down-to-earth individual who, faced with a career crisis that threatens the life of comfortable domestic affluence he has built for himself, succumbs with surprisingly few misgivings to an absurd New Age fix and gets more than he bargained for.

At heart *The Muse* is less a broadside against the industry than another of Brooks's subtly offbeat cautionary comedies of modern anxiety. Once again, a Me Generation everyman occupies an ideal lifestyle or system, blissfully unaware of its underlying precariousness. Whether it be the callow filmmaker's perfect experiment in documentary in *Real Life* (1979); the impossible fantasy of "true love" in *Modern Romance* (1981); the way a life of complacent materialism is exchanged for an equally deluded freedom of the road in the anti-Reagan-zeitgeist *Lost in America* (1985), or ended altogether by the ultimate bummer of sudden death at the start of *Defending Your Life* (1991), the Brooks protagonist is oblivious until too late. In *The Muse,* as in *Mother* (1996) and *Lost in America,* the great central comic conceit is the adoption of an improbable radical solution: when your marriage fails, move back in with your mother to figure out why your relationships with women don't work; when you don't get the promotion you feel you deserve, quit, drop out of society, and go on the road to find yourself; if your writing career goes south, hire a muse and do whatever she instructs, even if you can't shake the feeling that you're being shortchanged.

Brooks's protagonists tend to be successful yet average creative types who write or work in advertising or filmmaking (one of the incidental joys of *Modern Romance* is its dead accurate depiction of a film editor's working life). His characterizations effectively refract the contradictions, compromises, and neuroses of the Baby Boomer generation with its overdeveloped sense of entitlement and unapologetic materialism: narcissistic and controlling yet insecure and resigned, reflexively self-analytical yet lacking emotional self-honesty. It's hard to think of another American filmmaker who has dedicated himself or herself so completely to scrutinizing the foibles of his generational peers without becoming moralistic or sentimental.

Starting with his early-1970s bits for TV, his two unique records, *Comedy Minus One* (1973) and *A Star Is Bought* (1976), and his six short films for *Saturday Night Live* in 1975–76, his comic persona is smugly self-confident yet oblivious to his own absurdity. A number of his performances for other directors (starting out for Scorsese in *Taxi Driver* but notably in James L. Brooks's *Broadcast News* and *I'll Do Anything*) feed on the same persona, combining humbling misfortune with an ensuing struggle to overcome pervasive anxiety and regain existential terra firma.

But perhaps because of his sparse output as a feature director—seven films in twenty-five years—even some of Brooks's critical champions have called him an underachiever. I know what they mean. Brooks seems constitutionally incapable of going over the top in his performances and films, and he's not interested in blowing the audience away. In his elusive sui generis brand of antisentimental, observational comedy, the comic possibilities of character and situation are always restrained by a defining sense of plausible reality and authentic, self-revealing emotional experience. This places him completely at odds with American comedy's currently prevailing aesthetic—a parodic, cartoonish absurdism, fed on high energy, outrageous excess, and mock sentimentality—whose prime exponents include Jim Carrey, the Farrelly brothers, Ben Stiller, Will Farrell, and post–*Saturday Night Live* Adam Sandler and Mike Myers.

• • •

Are you sticking your neck out with The Muse, *a story about someone who faces rejection in Hollywood?*

I guess since that's what I've always done it doesn't feel so much like sticking my neck out. I've never come from a safe place; I sort of began my whole comedy career sticking my neck out. So I don't know any better. Hopefully, I'm always going to be honest enough with what I do where I can leave my neck out. I just don't consciously think in terms of safe and unsafe.

You don't feel there's a pattern in your work of exploring specific fears?

I think I do. I think that's the nature of writing. I don't think it would be fun to do it otherwise. Unless you do that, it doesn't get exciting. I've never made a sequel. I've never gone to a place that was familiar to me. I had seen lots of different movies about this town, and those scenes, to me, don't ring true. The people I've seen in other movies, cast as studio people or agents, they're just not what I believe is really there. I wanted a chance to put my two cents in. Casting Mark Feuerstein as opposed to Martin Short as the studio executive makes a big difference. I try not to do these parts in a clichéd way; I at least try to make them real enough that you don't even have to know about the business to know it's real.

Why is your work more rooted in realism than most current comedy?

Well, I didn't think about it like, "I'll do this and they'll do that." I once had an agent say to me, years ago—we were having some discussion over an argument about a studio project—and he said, "Gee, I don't know why you always take the hard road," and I said, "You think I see two roads?" You don't really analyze what you do, and if you stick around long enough, then maybe you'll start your own category, or you'll fit into a category.

When I started, one of the first things I ever did was *The Dean Martin Summer Show.* The producer, seeing one spot, gave me eight shows, and said to me, "Do you have material?" I said yes and I really didn't, and he said, "Okay, you'll start in four weeks." And I went home and figured out what kind of a comedian I would be, and I came back and showed him my stuff, and he said to me, "You know what? If you do this kind of material you're going to have trouble your whole life, because you're ten feet above the audience." I said, "I don't know what you're talking about—this is all I know how to do," and he took this long pause and said, "Okay, that was all I wanted to hear. Go do it." You just do what you know. Some people are right in the mainstream from the get-go. They don't ever have a problem with that, that's just who they are.

What inspired your film The Muse?

The idea of something or somebody that is going to sit on your shoulder and guide you through this stuff. It's so romantic and, obviously, it's such an important part of the history of creativity, this idea of a creative guardian angel. The movie certainly tells you that it's really in your head if you believe that it's true. I just always liked that idea that there was an outside party that could contribute to the success of a creative project. It's also the idea that Hollywood will embrace anybody and do it quickly. People rise up in this town very fast, and sometimes they're even criminals, let alone not who they say they are.

Do you think the character you play is a good screenwriter?

I think he's a good screenwriter going through the exact period that tons of screenwriters are. Ninety-nine percent of writers write for somebody. There're only a few people in life who ever get to write because they want to and people come to them. Most people write for hire. As those people get older, I think they all get a little scared when the executives become younger than their children; they get a little worried that they're not going to get those jobs anymore, so they start writing things that maybe they don't love or they're not close to. I think that's sort of what Steven Phillips [the character Brooks plays] is . . .

The distance between the character and you is probably greater than it's been in any of your other films.

People always like to think everything's you. I used to answer this question a lot—"*Lost in America,* is it you?" and I said, "I don't own a motorhome, I've never lost all my money in Las Vegas, I've never worked for an ad agency, but sure, why not?" I'm not interesting enough on my own that you'd want to see a film about me. My whole interest comes alive after I create something and can get it on its feet. Why would you want to see me sit in a room all day trying to do that? That's what Albert Brooks does.

But there is a kind of unspoken contract between you and the audience: You create something imaginary in its circumstances and they'll believe it's you up there.

I understand what you're saying, but let's go back to somebody like Jack Benny, one of the greatest radio and early television comedians that ever lived. The reason why he was so brilliant was that he did nothing. He would have these long, forty-second takes, where he would just stare. But the audience knew him so well that they laughed at those silences. He was known as someone who was cheap, the most frugal, he never paid his employees; this is what people roared at. One of the biggest laughs in the history of radio is: Jack Benny's walking home late at night and a guy comes out of an alley and says, "Your money or your life." And Benny doesn't say anything. And the audience starts laughing and laughing, and finally the guy says, "Your money or your life!" and Benny goes, "I'm thinking it over!"

His whole life, Jack Benny faced this: "Are you really that cheap?" And Jack Benny was one of the most charitable men that ever lived. These older comedians all played their own name. So it got confusing. I'm the last one to look at these characters that I play as being me. I've always hated the word "neurotic"—life is not an easy road for anybody, no matter who you are; so all I'm really doing is saying, "Look what happens."

When I was a kid, ninety-nine percent of the stand-up comedians just did jokes that had nothing to do with them and you could call them "everyman jokes." I don't know where it happened, but as stand-up comedy changed over the years, Everyman changed to Individual Man, and that's when I started. When I played Albert Brooks in *Real Life* I learned how confusing that gets, because people didn't know me very well then. I was reading reviews like, "This Albert Brooks should never be allowed to make another film, and he doesn't know how to handle a family. How dare he be so rough with children!" And I'm going, "Holy shit, don't people get it?" So, unless you play something so bizarre and unrealistic, you're always going to get mixed up with your work, which is just the way it is.

I would not have made *Modern Romance* unless I had that kind of trouble in my life with breaking up. I didn't do it as much as that character, but I did it enough to be able to write and do that, so for comedic purposes I take behavior that I might do and square it. And then you have a performance, you have a movie. You have to be fearless about it, you can't go, "Oh gee, am I gonna come off 'too this' or 'too that'?" Don't make the movie then, don't do that subject if that's what you're afraid of; play a lovable teddy bear. If I think about my next film and think, "This could be very embarrassing," I would never do it. You have to commit yourself to the part. If you don't do that, you have no chance of ever doing it great. I really did feel when *Real Life* came out that people would automatically go, "Oh, is he brilliant, the way he played that character with his own name!" And I was really surprised when that didn't happen. I saved the review that said, "Why would Paramount give this idiot the money to do such an important experiment?"

Which of your characters is closest to you, or the least removed?

They all had distances, and they all had similarities. Maybe that's too much of a safe answer, but it's really true. I don't think I could play a character that I didn't have something in common with. Maybe when I made *Modern Romance* I was closer to that kind of feeling than other feelings—no, I don't even think that's true. When I did *Defending Your Life* I was very consumed with the idea of fear and not being afraid. I still think about that subject. I think I'm equally invested in every movie. So the movies reflect what's going on in you and preoccupying you.

Yes, but because the movies take so long to make, [often] by the time the movie comes out you've dealt with that issue already. That must be weird.

It is weird. It's working in a time machine. When I went through that behavior that the character went through in *Modern Romance,* I was probably seventeen. I wasn't able to make movies then. But the behavior was so strong and interesting and weird that I stuffed it away so I could write about it.

When I made that movie, the studio had seen it lots of times with an audience, and they seemed to be fine; they were treating me nicely. Then they went up to San Francisco and tested it, and they just hated what they got, they didn't like those scores. And they treated me as if I had just made another movie than the one I had been showing them. They kept saying to me, "Add a psychiatrist scene," and I said, "Why?" And they said, "Explain that behavior, they don't understand what's wrong with him—listen to these cards: 'He's got a beautiful girl, a Porsche, what's his problem?'" I said, "You know what, I'm not being facetious, I don't know his problem. I can't explain it, I didn't write the movie as a philosopher, I just wrote it as someone showing the behavior." Now today I could give you that answer. I know this many years later, why people act like that. But I didn't know that then. And they just thought I was being an asshole.

Do you find the dialogue in your recent films reflects a more therapy-oriented sensibility?

I can't disagree with that. But that's just getting smarter. It's not something you leave in, or leave out on purpose. I just knew that one day I needed to write *Mother,* just having conversations with my mother for my whole life. I just found it so interesting, and I had never seen that put on film in that fashion.

Mother-son relationships tend to be depicted as somehow unhealthy, as in The Manchurian Candidate *or* Psycho.

Or they're weird, they're like John Candy and Maureen O'Hara [in the 1991 Chris Columbus film *Only the Lonely*]. I wanted an experience where I would go, "Oh my god, that's my mother, that's my mother's house, that's my mother's kitchen," and I knew I wasn't the only one. That movie had to have been more intellectualized than, say, *Real Life,* just in order to make it. The point of that movie, for that son to be able to reach a point where he could let his mother off the hook, that did need to be figured out. That's why people go to shrinks. So I did it in an hour and a half, where normally it would take you fifteen years.

I've read that you've always had a fascination with technology and science. In a number of your films, your characters come up with a perfect system or plan to solve their problems.

In *The Muse,* it's, "How do I get this person into my life to make everything okay?" Maybe in some unconscious way, I'm trying to put order to disorder. I've never said it that way before, but to me, that's funny. How do you order something that is not supposed to be ordered; how do you try to regiment your life where it's not supposed to be? The people who get into the biggest trouble are the ones who set up their cards the most carefully—those are the cards that fall the fastest. So here's a comedy character saying, "If I do A, B, and C, I'll get D," but he always gets F. In *Lost in America,* sitting down with Julie [Hagerty], telling her what it's going to be like if we have fifty-four grand, and we do this and do that, it's like a little computer spewing out these answers.

How do you think your filmmaking has evolved since you began?

You can't work at anything and not get a style, otherwise you'd be insane. You have to learn that there's no way to make your first film your third film. You just don't know what you don't know. I've learned how to do things for a budget. There was a time when I started to shoot with two cameras to speed things up. I just understand the constraints I've been given. I've learned about who to hire to help me, what kind of a crew I need to make it go fast and pleasant. It takes a while to learn the other crafts enough so that you can be intelligent about it. The first movie you ever do, if the cinematographer tells you he needs six hours to light a room and that's all there is to it, you have nothing to compare it to. Then when you see [cameraman] Michael Ballhaus do it in ten minutes and it looks brilliant, you now don't accept that any longer. That's the hardcore part of filmmaking.[1]

There's a real sense of control and ease in how you cover scenes. It doesn't feel as though you do lots of setups; you seem to know what you want.

Yes, I do. There's a couple of scenes in *The Muse* that I'm really proud of because they're exquisitely simple. When Sharon Stone and Andie MacDowell have that first lunch together, that's one very slow move; it starts on one side of the table, featuring one of the characters a little bit, and moves to the other. It was designed that way, we worked hard to make it that way, that was important to me. I think I have a style I am very intent on—I've always sort of imagined movies as people looking through a window. Sort of peeping in on the goings-on. So unless it's for a comedic effect, I don't make the camera the star.

In scenes in restaurants or public places you'll cut to a single of an incidental character like a waiter or a store clerk for a moment, giving emphasis to someone we never see again.

I think that's one of the most fun parts of movies. One of the best reviews of *Lost in America* I got was from Pauline Kael: she said the little characters that come and go in his movie are like candy for the audience. I love little characters. The more interesting they can be, the better.

So the casting process must be a really important part of directing for you.

It's absolutely crucial. One of the funniest scenes in *The Muse* is the Italian guy in the Spago party [Mario Opinato]. There was only so much I could write. So I saw forty people who had dialects, and sat in my office with them and tried to play. And this was the one guy who never dropped the ball. Whatever I asked him, he came back at me, and I just knew something could happen. And when we got on the set where there were multiple cameras—we just went. Generally, I don't like to ad-lib in movies. If the opportunity arises and you have somebody who's capable, you can maybe take a little bit from [the script]. But what never works is where you don't know where to go and you start to make it up, it looks made up. In this case, this guy was wonderful. Any ball I threw him, he just threw it back.

When you're casting a role that's going to play opposite you, do you read with the actors?

Absolutely. People say, "How can you direct yourself if you act?" Well, there's one aspect of it that's easier, because you're right there looking into their eyes. If it's false, you can tell as an actor it's not going. That's one thing that makes one director different from another. That's all it really is, is how you feel that person should be, how I feel that person should be, how Jim Carrey feels that person should be.

Another question about cinematic style: you favor a consistently sweeping, symphonic score that is not particularly fashionable.

Well, I'm a musical person and I have these notes in my head. I gave Elton John [the composer of *The Muse*'s score] a temp score of classical music, which I never gave any other composer before. I always like the juxtaposition—trying to do the film with the action and characters as real-seeming as they could be, and then cushioning it in a sort of a classical musical sense with more of a timeless movie feel to it. Is it ironic?

I don't know that it's irony, but it might be.

In *Real Life,* when the psychology consultant quits, suddenly this music comes in. Up until then we've been watching the film as it's being shot, but at that moment we realize that the film has been edited and even scored. The director is in the cutting room making decisions.

I had a lot of scenes in *Real Life* that never got in the movie, and one of them was a scene with me and Mort Lindsey talking about what the [musical score] would be. I was sitting in an office with him, and I had pictures of [Charles] Grodin up on the wall, and he was at the piano looking at Grodin trying to come up with a theme, and I kept saying, "That's no good, that's no good, that's too sad."

How did you meet your writing collaborator Monica Johnson,[2] and how do you work together?

She was familiar with my stand-up, and Penny Marshall was friends with both of us, and [Monica] said, "I want to meet this guy," and we hit it off.

And except for *Defending Your Life*, I've been working with her ever since. We sit together, I talk into a tape recorder, so I do the main babbling, and Monica will throw in anything that she thinks of, say something in a way she wants to say it. *Modern Romance* we wrote in a car, with a tape recorder on. I'm the one who's doing the primary; I play all the parts and the stage direction, and Monica has all the ideas and lines she can think of. She provides this place where comedy can live, she's very muselike in that sense. From the very beginning, when you talk about the Albert Brooks character, she's understood that character very innately. Not me, him. She understands that guy very well. It was a challenge for me to do it without her, it was harder. It's much nicer to work with somebody, it's more fun.

So you're each other's first audience?

Yes, absolutely. In other words, I know if I can't make Monica laugh it won't go any further than that.

Do you have a sense of what need your work satisfies in you?

Well, up until recently, when I found my wife and I had a child, it was almost the only thing I did. And I don't know what else I would have been, or why I'm even living, if not. I just had to get all this stuff out. From the beginning, especially if you're funny from such a young age, you almost have to do it, or you go insane.

Did being considered a prodigy and comic genius create pressure?

It's a great thing, and it can be a burden. If you get clogged up with that shit, you can be in bad trouble. The worst thing that can happen to anybody trying to be creative is to feel, "Oh my god, I'm not living up to something." To me, the people that seem to be rewarded the most, who are in creative work, are the people who stay in the longest. Just stick in there, and keep doing and doing. I turned down four movies that Tom Hanks took early in our careers, including *Bachelor Party* (1984) and *Dragnet* (1987). I was there going, "Oh my god, my reputation. I can't do that." I don't think Tom Hanks thought like that, and you can't be in a better place in terms of respect than he is right now. So if you do get bogged down with who you are, it's not good.

Was there a point when that did get on top of you?

Yes. Absolutely. I still feel it. I still make my decisions based on somebody I want to respect. There was a time where television was the worst thing you could ever do. That doesn't seem to be true anymore, and many of the things that I still hold on to, quite frankly, I don't even think are true. But they're still true for me. I was trying to live up to something that I wanted to be. But you have to do that to have a career that you are proud of. It's unhealthy where it keeps you from doing something you might have fun at. You can make some mistakes and have fun doing them, and you're gonna turn out okay. But there was a time in my life where I thought if I made one mistake it was one mistake too many.

One experience that really taught me a lot was *The Scout*. Monica and I rewrote this script. The movie we wrote ended in a completely different way. It did not end like *Rocky* (1976), with that bullshit big ending. The way that movie ended was, he was taken down to the field, he threw one pitch, and the movie was over. He just was able to let the ball go. It was a very gentle, quiet moment, where you just knew that kid was going to be all right. And the studio made [director] Michael Ritchie put on this ending, and I got so upset. They tested it with both endings, and it tested nine points higher with the phony ending. I remember I was doing the press junket in New York and the *Times* said, "Albert Brooks should be ashamed, it's the worst ending." I'm happy that was the only one of those in my life.

Why didn't you direct The Scout?

I didn't want to. I really only did *The Scout* because I just wanted to play that part. I liked that character, a guy who traveled around—it was like *Death of a Salesman*. I didn't want to direct a baseball movie. A lonely type of guy to play, but I guess it was the first at-bat. That script was originally written for Rodney Dangerfield; it was lying around, never going to get made, and I said I would like to do that. And that sort of got it alive, and then it really needed a rewrite because it was written very silly. It had no reality to it at all. It's very rare that artists get to hold out for what they want. I got spoiled. Even if it meant I couldn't make an expensive movie, or I couldn't make them as often as I wanted, there's no movie with my name on it that I am not proud of and cannot say this is the way I wanted it to be.

Does it seem to you now that directing was always the natural destination for you?

I still like to act. I enjoy acting in projects that I don't direct. Basically, I wound up directing because I could never find anybody else to do it. From the very beginning it was clear to me that my comedy had to get me to do it.

If I gave *Real Life* to Carl Reiner it wouldn't have been *Real Life,* it would have been another movie. That's what directing is. Directing is simply all the choices, and if I think you're the best person to play [a part], and the other director thinks Brad Pitt's the best person, well, there's the different movie right there. So it starts there and goes to every decision there is. Should he live in a two-story house? No! He should live in a bad apartment.

So you've got to do it. It forces you. And certainly, once I wrote, I had to direct. If I never wrote a word I never would have been a director. It's carrying out the instructions correctly, and it would have been way more frustrating standing on the side going, "Oh, don't do it like that!" On *The Scout* I never told Michael Ritchie what to do, but there were many times where I had to leave because I thought, "Gee, I wouldn't have Brendan [Fraser] do it that way . . ." But that wasn't my job, and I'm not that kind of person. I don't butt in like that.

If you had to give up two of them, which one would you keep: acting, directing, writing?

If I had to, if I was forced, like it was Russia? I feel I would like to keep acting. That's the way I feel right now, but I don't want to give up any of them. I feel I'm entering an age where there's a shitload of parts that I could really play, and I'd like to keep doing that. Now, talk to me in a year. The hardest of the three is writing. It's the most gratifying; also the toughest. I would act in someone else's movie, I might even direct a movie that I hadn't written, but I'd never write a movie and that would be it. That I just wouldn't do. It would be too difficult.

Given that, does your talent as a whole lie in your writing side, or in your performing?

I know when I'm writing, I'm acting out the different people, so I would say my acting ability has helped everything. And the reason actors like working for me as a director is that I do really understand what they do, and they feel comfortable. I'm not looking at them like, "Who are you and why do you get paid so much?"

So writing and directing are manifestations of yourself as a performer.

If there were fifty great parts for me when I was twenty or twenty-five, I probably never would have done this, but out of necessity I had to do it. I wasn't getting anything. If I was able to get a lot of work as a young actor I never would have had the discipline to write and direct.

Before you began your career, you aspired to be a serious actor and studied acting at Carnegie-Mellon. Why did you go in that direction when it was already established that you had this natural gift for making people laugh?

In that era, the late '60s, there was nobody in stand-up; the profession of stand-up was just Vegas and cigars and the Friars Club and Sheckey Greene—it wasn't a cool thing to do. If you wanted to work, you had to go work and live in Vegas. My father was a famous radio comedian,[3] and I had certainly seen that part of it. I just didn't have any fascination or desire to do stand-up comedy. I always wanted to act, and at Carnegie I got a lot of shows my freshman year. I left after a year and a half. I also went to L.A. City College for a year and did the same thing.

What particularly stayed with you?

There was a guy named Tom Hill who taught the most wonderful thing of all, and that was the economy of acting. We get back to Jack Benny and how less is more. That always made a lot of sense to me.

What happened when you returned to L.A.?

I came back here and tried to get work, and I was nineteen, and nobody at nineteen was getting much acting. Whenever a part would come up, Richard Dreyfuss would get it. I had this man at the William Morris office who has basically been in my life ever since, Herb Nanas, and I'd always go and make these people laugh. One of my friends, Larry Bishop, whose father was Joey Bishop, had a ventriloquist hanging around. I picked it up, and one thing led to another, and I created "Danny and Dave," and it made everybody laugh. These people convinced me—and they were wrong, by the way—but they said, "Listen, if you'll be willing to be funny, you'll get everything you ever want, you will zoom right past everybody else and get right to the front of the casting door." Well, I didn't; what I did was get a lot of stand-up comedy work. I probably got *Taxi Driver* because Marty Scorsese was a fan of my comedy. But it took too long to get that one part.

I started in reverse. I did all of my starting on national television. I'd think up these bits, I'd go down to *The Dean Martin Show* or *Ed Sullivan* and do it for the first time, and then after three or four years of that I put together an hour and opened for Neil Diamond. So, I went the opposite way.

How would you characterize the comic sensibility that you shared and helped shape?

I think the answer is that it was acting comedy. It was taking what I really wanted to do and putting it in the stand-up world. I would play these characters. Most of your stand-up comedians were not actors—they were joke tellers. On my first record, *Comedy Minus One,* one side of it was twenty-five minutes from my stand-up act that I was currently doing, and that was talking to the audience. But on television I would never do that. I certainly wasn't going to do, "Two Jews walk into a bar . . ." so I started out satirizing show business, the very bullshit part of show business that I hated. I did these entertainers that were terrible at it and didn't know it. That's the whole nature of making fun of the beast, to punch it in the mouth and see where it goes. You do it to tear it down. There were guys my age, and there still are people who are twenty years old, who can stand up with a cigar and tell jokes. That will never go away.

When you acted in Taxi Driver, *did you have any idea how it would turn out?*

No, I really didn't. I had waited so long to make a start that I would come up to Marty occasionally and say, "Do you think this is going to help me as an actor?" I think it's very rare that people who wind up doing something that lasts have an idea of that, because if you do have an idea of that, then you're sort of out of the moment.

I'd heard that your role was expanded once you started working.

It wasn't even there. One of the funniest lines anyone's ever said to me was at the wrap party. Paul Schrader [the screenwriter of *Taxi Driver*] comes up to me and says, "I just want to thank you. This was the one guy I didn't know." I'm thinking, "Jesus Christ, you've got a movie filled with murderers and pimps, all I'm doing is working in a campaign office—this is the guy you didn't know?!" The way we worked (I don't know if Marty continues to work like this) was, we would improvise during rehearsals, and he would tape those. Then he would commit the best of that to the script, and that's what he would shoot. So, he really didn't like you making it up the day the camera was rolling. It occurred to me that if you work in a campaign office, one of the things that would be your job is to get boxes of twenty thousand buttons. So I made up this phone conversation about the "We are the People" badges and being upset.

What contribution did you make to shaping your character in Broadcast News?

The arc of the character was pretty clear as written: this character needed to have a catastrophic moment where he failed, [but] in the early stages Jim

[Brooks] was not sure what should happen. I had that luxury of talking to Jim as he was writing, which is a great thing if you can do that with the writer. I remember, at eleven-thirty at night, seeing this man on CNN have that flop-sweat experience, and I called up Jim and said, "Turn on the television!" So that was sort of how the sweating happened.

What about your work in I'll Do Anything?

I wish you could have seen the musical [version]. That was the greatest thing in the world, and it broke my heart that the movie came out like it did. The irony of that movie is, the very thing it was about is what it succumbed to. I mean, here's a movie whose whole being is about testing and succumbing to the testing, and that's exactly what happened to Jim. I understand why, but the ambition was so great, if he had stuck to it, in my opinion, it certainly wouldn't have done any worse, and in the long run it would have been a really important movie.

Did you do a good job with the singing and dancing?

You weren't going to buy my albums and make out to them, but I was sort of in the Rex Harrison vein. I sold a song, and I did it within the character. I had the title song, "I'll Do Anything." People were lined up to see the preview of that terrible movie that my character produced, and he was doing up and down the line singing, "I'll do anything to make you like me." And then there was a song called "There Is Lonely," after he got the opening weekend grosses; it was so funny to sing that kind of song to that subject. We worked a solid year. As I look back, I got to study with Twyla Tharp, who did the choreography. Where would I have ever gotten that chance? That was a thrill.

Is it true your character was modeled on producer Joel Silver?

Well, he never spoke to me again, so it must have been.

August 1999

ALBERT BROOKS (1947–)

1979 *Real Life* (Albert Brooks). Director, co-script, actor.
1981 *Modern Romance* (Albert Brooks). Director, co-script, actor.
1985 *Lost in America* (Albert Brooks). Director, co-script, actor.
1991 *Defending Your Life* (Albert Brooks). Director, script, actor.
1994 *The Scout* (Michael Ritchie). Co-script, actor.

1996 *Mother* (Albert Brooks). Director, co-script, actor.

1999 *The Muse* (Albert Brooks). Director, co-script, actor.

2005 *Looking for Comedy in the Muslim World* (Albert Brooks). Director, script, actor.

Actor only in *Taxi Driver* (1976); *Private Benjamin* (1980); *Twilight Zone: The Movie* (1983); *Terms of Endearment* (voice, 1983); *Unfaithfully Yours* (1984); *Broadcast News* (1987); *I'll Do Anything* (1994); *Critical Care* (1997); *Doctor Doolittle* (voice, 1998); *Out of Sight* (1998); *My First Mister* (2001); *The In-Laws* (2003); *Finding Nemo* (voice, 2003); *The Simpsons Movie* (voice, 2007).

Television acting in *Hot Wheels* (voice, 1969 series); *The Odd Couple* (1970 episodes); *Love, American Style* (1971 episodes); *The New Dick Van Dyke Show* (1972 episode); *Saturday Night Live* (1975 episodes); *The Simpsons* (various episodes); and *Weeds* (2008 episodes).

Television standup comedy appearances include *Dean Martin Presents the Golddiggers* (1968); *The Dean Martin Show* (1970); *The Everly Brothers Show* (1970); *The Ed Sullivan Show* (1970); *The David Frost Show* (1971); *The Golddiggers* (1971); *The Flip Wilson Show* (1972); *The Tonight Show* (multiple appearances); and *Saturday Night Live* (multiple appearances).

Television writing and/or directing credits include contributions to episodes of *Saturday Night Live* (1975–76).

NOTES

1 Michael Ballhaus started out his illustrious career closely associated with the New German Cinema's Rainer Werner Fassbinder. Ballhaus has worked prolifically in America since the early 1980s, including as Martin Scorsese's cinematographer on several acclaimed films. He also shot *Broadcast News* and *I'll Do Anything*.

2 Monica Mcgowan Johnson, who has collaborated with Brooks on the screenplays of six films to date, started out in television working on the *Mary Tyler Moore Show* and *Laverne and Shirley* series. Apart from her Albert Brooks films, Johnson has also written *Americathon* (1979) and *Jekyll and Hyde . . . Together Again* (1982). Since this interview was originally published, Brooks also wrote the solo script for *Looking for Comedy in the Muslim World*.

3 Brooks's father was old-time radio comedian Harry Parke; his mother was actress Thelma Leeds.

INTERVIEW BY **MIKAEL COLVILLE-ANDERSEN**

JEAN-CLAUDE CARRIÈRE BREAKING THE RULES

Jean-Claude Carrière's working relationship with Luis Buñuel produced six film classics, and he went on to write *The Tin Drum* (1979), *The Unbearable Lightness of Being* (1988), *Valmont* (1989), *Cyrano de Bergerac* (1990), and many other films—over one hundred in all—in several languages (including English). In the year 2000 he became the only non–U.S. citizen ever honored by the Writers Guild of America with its Laurel Award for lifetime achievement.

Not content with merely writing, Carrière has served as an unofficial dean of French film, written books on film and screenwriting, and hosted a debate program on French television.

He is the thinking man's screenwriter, well known for his philosophizing over not only particular screenplays but film in general. His relationship with Buñuel figures prominently in his career. Indeed, the collaboration between the two men, which began over a common love of wine, developed into one of the most prolific in European film history.

Well-versed and well-spoken, Carrière is an old hand at interviews and the source of countless nuggets of wisdom and anecdotes.

• • •

It could interesting to hear from you how you got started in the film industry as a screenwriter.

Well, I started as a novelist, as so many did back then. I wrote a novel at twenty-three and my publisher had a contract with Jacques Tati, the French film director, to publish novels based on his films. I took part in a contest, with two or three other novelists, where we had to write a chapter, like an essay, as a trial. Tati chose my chapter. He was very famous at the time and when I visited him in his production office near the Champs-Elysées,

I was very young—twenty-four and still a student—but we got on quite well. I wrote two short stories: one from *Mr. Hulot's Holiday* (*Les vacances de Monsieur* Hulot, 1953) and one from *Mon oncle* (1958).

Through my contact with Jacques Tati, I met many other people. One of them was Pierre Etaix, who was Tati's assistant, and Etaix and I started writing short films. But four or five years went by as I had to do my military service—there was a war in Algeria—and when I returned I was almost thirty. By chance we met a producer who wanted to do some short films. We did two of them in 1961 with both of us co-writing and co-directing. So, I started as a novelist and as a director.

The second of these shorts, *Heureux anniversaire* (1962), won the Academy Award in Hollywood. We didn't even know what it was. The producer told us we got the Oscar and we said, "What's the Oscar?" After that he gave us the opportunity to write and direct a feature film. This film, called *The Suitor* (*Le soupirant*, 1962), won the Prix de Luc in France. It was very successful. However, I had chosen not to be co-director and to be solely the screenwriter because I had some other possibilities to write books and perhaps work in the theater. I didn't want to commit myself totally to film direction. Once you have succeeded in becoming a film director you can't do anything else. You are a sort of prisoner in a—hopefully—golden cage. Not always, you know.

When you are a screenwriter, you are just a screenwriter, even if you collaborate with the director, but you can keep publishing books, novels, essays, and become a playwright. Which I did, a few years later, and have since been working with Peter Brook [the English theater director] for twenty-four years, as well as writing several other plays.

So that was a sort of crossroads, at the very beginning of my career. When people ask me why I'm not a film director, that is my answer. Also, I believe I am less gifted as a film director than as a screenwriter—which doesn't mean I believe I'm gifted as a screenwriter—but to be a director you have to have what we call in French an *idée fixe.* A sort of obsession to think every day and every hour of every day about the film you are going to make. For two, three, four years. To get obsessed about what you are preparing.

I'm not that type. I'm very much disposed. I often go from one project to another, and sometimes I work on two different things simultaneously. And that is absolutely bad for a director. I didn't know that at the beginning. I am speaking in retrospect now that I know a bit about what my life has been like. When you're twenty-five or thirty it is impossible to say what your life will be like. It is much easier to talk about it when you are sixty-eight. But I can see clearly now that I probably made the right decision.

Interesting that you came into film from a literary background. Where did you go from there?

Immediately after *The Suitor,* by Etaix, I met Luis Buñuel. That was in 1963. He was looking for a French co-writer as he was going to direct a film in French. That was *Diary of a Chambermaid* (*Le journal d'une femme de chambre,* 1964), based on the French novel and to be shot in France. He met with three or four "young" screenwriters and he, again, chose me like Jacques Tati had done. Buñuel chose me only after eating lunch together and getting me to talk about the possible adaptation of the book. So, I went to Spain to work with one of the greatest directors of the era, a man whom I deeply admired. I was very impressed at the beginning. That started a collaboration which last for almost twenty years. We wrote nine scripts together, six of which became Buñuel's films and we even wrote a book, *My Last Breath* or *My Last Sigh,* depending on whether you are American or English.

So that was about it. I went on to write for many other directors but the first two were Pierre Etaix and Buñuel. Buñuel was extremely faithful to me. I had no reason to refuse but he constantly came to me to work with him again.

Your relationship with Buñuel is well documented. While it is clear what the collaboration gave to you, what do you think you gave to Buñuel? How did your influence affect him and his filmmaking?

That I cannot answer, apart from one point. Without me and without Serge Silberman, the producer, perhaps Buñuel would not have made so many films after he was sixty-five. We really encouraged him to work. That's for sure. Now about what we did together, the quality or no quality of our work, I don't know. But it was a very close relationship. We were always alone in some remote place, often in Mexico or Spain, talking French and Spanish, without friends, without women, without wives. Absolutely no one around. Just the two of us. Eating together, working together, drinking together to get absolutely obsessed about the script we were working on. I calculated that we ate together, just the two of us, more than two thousand times. Which is much more than many couples can say.

So it was a very close relationship and nobody can say that one gave an idea to the other. There are only a few things I could mention. At the very beginning, and this goes for many screenwriters who work with a master, I was so thrilled, so happy, so impressed that I was ready to love any idea from Buñuel. Whenever he told me something I always said, "It's wonderful, let's do it!" Always killing my own critical instinct and restraining from suggesting my own ideas about the adaptation.

After two or three weeks, Serge Silberman came down from Paris to Madrid, where we were working. He invited me out to dinner, without Buñuel, which was rather unusual. We always ate together, the three of us. So, after a long dinner and talking about French politics or whatever, he told me something. He said, "Luis is very happy with you. You work a lot and are a hard worker. But . . . you must say 'no' to him from time to time." I found out later that Buñuel had asked Silberman to come down from Paris to tell me this one thing. That I had to oppose him. If not, my contribution was only fifty percent of what it could be. In that type of collaboration, when two people work so closely together on a common work, it is absolutely necessary that one is not the slave of the other—based on fame, age, power. No, you must try to be equal. Which is quite difficult.

So, from then on, I tried from time to time to say no. To oppose. To say, "Luis, I don't like this idea." At times, Buñuel was a bit irritated, but generally he was happy about it. During the writing of the second film, *Belle de jour* (1967), we almost reached a real sense of collaboration.

There was another type of collaboration with Buñuel. Buñuel had a type of surreal, I would say, tendency, or inclination, and I did as well. We were never rational. When he made *An Andalusian Dog* (*Un chien andalou*, 1929), his first film with Salvador Dali, they had one rule. The rule was that when one of them proposed an idea the other had three seconds, no more, to say yes or no. They didn't want the brain to intervene. They wanted an instinctive reaction coming, hopefully, from their subconscious. We used this process often although it was not easy. When you propose something you always want to explain your reasons for why you proposed this or that. And that must be—you know—put aside. It is a very difficult way of working. It requires a very alert mind to constantly be creative and invent and find new things to propose, all without becoming exhausted. Gradually, step by step, you discover, and I'm quoting Buñuel here, that the human imagination is a muscle that can be trained and developed like memory. It is one of the faculties of the brain that knows no limits. If I learned one thing from Buñuel, that would be it.

Working with Tati and Etaix I had learned how to observe the reality around us. Watching people, which really is a difficult task, and how to listen. In the streets, in the bars, in the cafés, on the metro. All my life, every day, I go to cafés and ride the metro—watching, listening and taking notes. I draw sketches of what reality gives me to nourish me. Of course that kind of reality has to be developed, transformed, elaborated on. I would say sixty percent of my work with Tati and Etaix was doing just that: sitting at cafés observing people, contemplating, trying to find a story for every passer-by and every couple. To listen to phrases and conversations, to take note of gestures, to record things that reveal something about the characters. Buñuel was also a great observer but he taught me how to use the imagination within first. How to look deep down inside ourselves in any given situation and to take it as far as possible.

The key word would be exploration. To explore all the different possibilities.

You wrote about the "Vanishing Screenplay" in your book The Secret Language of Film. *There is one thing I have been wondering about. You are one of the most well-known screenwriters but by and large the screenwriter, especially in Europe, is an invisible species. How do you feel about the anonymous role of the screenwriter in the film process?*

There is a certain paradox about the role of the screenwriter. He has to work as hard as possible, to give everything he has, only to build up someone else's work. He has to know that from the very beginning. He is a collaborator. He is not working on his own film but on a common work. The master, most of the time, is the director. Sometimes the actor—the star—but very rarely the screenwriter. He must know that. If he cannot accept that it is best that he chooses not to be a screenwriter. Except if he writes for television, which is often different.

Once I was in Venice with Peter Fleischmann, a German director, with a film. There were three hundred people in the cinema to hear us speak. Peter asked them, "You are all involved in the film industry in one way or another. Who can name the director of *Dallas?*" Nobody could. So, in some cases, the name of the director is just as anonymous as the name of the screenwriter. The star is the series itself. Or the characters, or the actors. In television, the role of the screenwriter is the same as that of the director. We don't know, at least in France, the stars among the TV directors.

The fame of the film director was really established in the '50s, '60s, and '70s. But since the '80s, the great masters—Stanley Kubrick is the most recent one to have disappeared—have all gone. Now, if you consider the active film industries in France, England, Denmark, or many European countries, the director has become much more anonymous than he used to be in the past. This is dangerous in a way because the film risks lacking a real personality.

My way, and I don't recommend this to everybody, has been to work closely with the director. Even if the director tells me that he is not a writer, an author, I need him to be there in front of me when I tell him what I want to do, or read some of the scenes for him. When I worked with Buñuel, Pierre Etaix, Milos Forman, Louis Malle, Volker Schlöndorff, the director was a co-writer. If the director is not a co-writer, I still need him to be around. I need to go to him, to talk with him, to look at research material with him, to talk about the film.

My opinion is that the work of the screenwriter is the beginning of the film adventure. It is not the end of a literary adventure. On the contrary. The screenwriter is a filmmaker. He doesn't work on a written process. The written word is very temporary. It is going to vanish and disappear and be thrown away at the end of the shooting. He is working on a film, so he had better work with the one who is making the film, in order to reach the point where they are working on the same film. That is the key phrase. Sometimes, after two or three weeks I have realized that we are working on two different films. That we see the film in two completely different ways. That is tragic. That will end in failure.

We must get as close as possible as soon as possible, and for as long as possible. There are many ways to do it. You can make drawings. For instance, you are sitting there in front of me right now. Imagine you are the director and I am the screenwriter. Your left side is my right side. And your right is my left. Already, we are not in the same film space. If I say to you, "The mother enters on the right side," your right and mine are different. So together we have to reach a third space—the film's space—and move constantly around, not in your space or in mine, but in the third space. We have to check it all the time that we see the same image all the time. That is absolutely vital.

In order to reach that invented third space you need to make drawings. I drew hundreds of scenes for Buñuel. It was really a necessity. At night, when I was alone, I would draw some quick sketches of the scenes we had been working on that day. The next day I would ask Buñuel, without showing him the sketches, for example, "In the scene with the paratroopers," from *The Discreet Charm of the Bourgeoisie* (*Le charme discret de la bourgeoisie*, 1972), "from which side do they enter?" If he said, "From the right," I would look at my sketch and if we had both pictured the right side, I knew we were in the same space, the same film.

The same applies for the sound and for the tone of the dialogue, which is easier because we are already beginning to act it out and improvise. It works sometimes with the rhythm of the film, which is also very important to establish. If one of the two is working on a fast-paced film and the other on a slow one—tragic. Failure. Disaster.

All these points are important in establishing the conditions for a good collaboration. The most difficult point is not to try to force your status on the other. To dictate your power. To win. To gain something. Not at all. However, it is difficult not to fall into that trap. It is human to say, "I want to be right." And to be right I am willing to say absurd things. Idiotic things, in order to impose my point of view. In a long-term collaboration, like with Buñuel or Peter Brook, the three-second rule is a very good exercise. Excellent. It reveals a lot of things about yourself.

You wrote in The Secret Language of Film *that there have never been enough screenwriters. However, nowadays, more and more people are saying that they want to write for films as opposed to directing. What can these people do to become screenwriters? Where is the inspiration for writing for film?*

Writing for films requires a know-how, a technical knowledge. You have to know how a film gets made. If you don't, there is no point in writing. I have never, in my whole life, seen a script written by an amateur, regardless of their talent, become a film. Never. It's never happened. You know, the unsolicited scripts you receive in the post. It's never happened. I've never seen one example. The only way to become a professional screenwriter is to get onto a team. To get into contact with a group of people who make films, preferably of the same generation at the beginning. Like I did with Pierre Etaix and like all the people I have known have done. Become a part of a group and start from there. Not a writer who delivers a script to a bunch of technicians. That is fatal. That is a lethal literary attitude.

The best way to become a screenwriter is to participate humbly in the making of a film. To sit there and see how the camera is being used, how the lights are arranged. To sit there and see how a script, not your own script—somebody else's—is being transformed during the magical process of shooting. The transfer from paper to film. That is absolutely essential. You have to know that what you write is not written to be published. It is written to be forgotten and to be transformed into something else. Into another kind of matter. Absolutely essential. That is the best way.

Then, of course, it is necessary to have ideas. The work of a screenwriter is not only to write a film and to know all about the technical side of things:

the sound, the images, the editing. His work, his function, is to look for new ideas. That is very important. To be able to offer a bouquet of different ideas. Not only one. A novelist is very often a man or woman who has written one book. A very personal tale which they offer to a publisher. If the publisher says no, they take it to another publisher. That is not the case with the screenwriter. I'm speaking from my own experience and not trying to generalize. There may be exceptions.

But to me the role of the screenwriter is a double one. To look for ideas—by reading the papers, listening to things you hear in the street, having an idea form in your imagination—and to write it down in two or three pages, no more, so as not to forget it. That should be a part of your everyday life. That is your function in society; to look for stories for the cinema. Then when one of these stories is chosen by a producer and a director to become a film with your help, it is absolutely necessary to be able to go deeper into the story and remain on the same technical level as the director.

Many, many novelists fail when they try to become screenwriters because they really believe that writing for a film is writing. It's not. Writing for a film is filming.

What do you think about all the screenwriting books that have appeared on the bookshelves? Most of them American and writing about Hollywood structure and abiding by the three-act structure and plot points and what have you. Are these books of any use to the screenwriter?

Well, I know Syd Field very well. He's been here many times and we've had long talks about this. I think these books are useful. I find them very boring to read but they are useful in one aspect. You must betray them. You mustn't follow them too closely. You must know the rules before you can break them. If not, you will always repeat the same structure.

These books often talk about building up a story, building a structure, and this is useful to know but only you are capable of not doing it and knowing when not to do it. Or to do something else. It's a very ancient and philosophical attitude. Kant said the same thing, not about screenwriting *[laughs]*, but about any kind of law. If you want to break the laws, you have to know them first. And know them very, very well. So, these books are useful as long as you don't obey.

One of the dangers of American cinema is to constantly make the same film while the world is changing. A *Frankenstein* remake, another Batman film and so on. All the classical themes. Another point which I discussed with [Ingmar] Bergman once is the fact that many films are now shown on television. The TV market has become very important over the past twenty-five years. It forces the writers and directors to "hook" the audience at the very beginning of the film. This was never the case in the classical cinema in the '30s and '40s and even the '50s. The classical cinema back then inherited a great deal from classical theater in the nineteenth century. It very often began with what we call in French *la scène d'exposition*—an exposition scene without action. Now, if you start a film on television with ten minutes of slow dialogue just to explain where we are and what's going to happen and who is who, people have already switched to another channel.

So the rules are never forever. The rules are changing all the time depending on society, on the evolution of people, of nations, of the way of life. As well as the way of thinking. It also depends very much on the new ways of releasing films and novels and what have you. And the Internet, that's another thing. All the new possibilities for releasing films digitally will no doubt change, covertly, the way films are written.

In which way?

[Smiles.] We don't know yet. We never know anything beforehand but we have to be prepared to know and to learn.

October 1999

JEAN-CLAUDE CARRIÈRE (1931–)

1961 *Rupture* (Pierre Etaix). Co-script (short film).

1962 *Heureux anniversaire* (Pierre Etaix). Co-producer, co-script (short film).

Le soupirant (Pierre Etaix). Co-script.

1964 *Le journal d'une femmme de chambre / Diary of a Chambermaid* (Luis Buñuel). Co-script.

1965 *Viva Maria!* (Louis Malle). Co-script.

Yoyo (Pierre Etaix). Co-script.

Le bestiaire d'amour (Gérald Calderon). Script (documentary).

1966 *Tant qu'on a la santé* (Pierre Etaix). Co-script.

Hotel Paradiso (Peter Glenville). Co-script.

Cartes sur table (Jesus Franco). Co-story, script.

Miss Muerte (Jesus Franco). Co-story, script.

1967 *Belle de jour* (Luis Buñuel). Co-script.

Le voleur / The Thief of Paris (Louis Malle). Co-script.

1968 *Pour un amour lointain* (Edmon Séchan). Co-script.

1969 *La pince à ongles* (Jean-Claude Carrière). Director, co-script.

La voie lactée / The Milky Way (Luis Buñuel). Co-script.

La piscine (Jacques Deray). Co-dialogue, co-adaptation.

Le grand amour (Pierre Etaix). Co-script.

1970 *Borsalino* (Jacques Deray). Co-script.

1971 *Taking Off* (Milos Forman). Co-script.

L'alliance (Christian de Chalonge). Script, based on Carrière's own novel.

Un peu de soleil dans l'eau froide (Jacques Deray). Dialogue, co-adaptation.

1972 *Le charme discret de la bourgeoisie / The Discreet Charm of the Bourgeoisie* (Luis Buñuel). Co-script.

Liza (Marco Ferreri). Co-dialogue, co-script.

Le droit d'aimer (Eric Le Hung). Co-script.

Le moine (Adonis Kyrou). Co-script.

Un homme est mort (Jacques Deray). Co-script.

1974 *Le fantôme de la liberté / The Phantom of Liberty* (Luis Buñuel). Co-script.

Dorotheas Rache (Peter Fleischmann). Co-script.

Un amour de pluie (Jean-Claude Brialy). Uncredited contribution.

France société anonyme (Alain Comeau). Co-script.

Grandeur nature (Luis García Berlanga). Dialogue.

La femme aux bottes rouges (Juan Luis Buñuel). Co-script.

1975 *La chair de l'orchidée* (Patrice Chéreau). Co-script.

La faille (Peter Fleischmann). Co-script.

Leonor (Juan Luis Buñuel). Co-script.

Sérieux comme le plaisir (Robert Benayoun). Co-script.

1976 *Les oeufs brouillés* (Jöel Santoni). Co-script.

1977 *Cet obscur objet du désir / That Obscure Object of Desire* (Luis Buñuel). Co-script.

Le diable dans la boîte (Pierre Lary). Co-script.

Le gang (Jacques Deray). Co-script.

Juliet pot de colle (Philippe de Broca). Script.

1978 *Un papillon sur l'épaule* (Jacques Deray). Co-script.
Chaussette surprise (Jean-François Davy). Co-script.

1979 *Die blechtromme / The Tin Drum* (Volker Schlöndorff). Co-script.
Slachtvee (Patrick Conrad). Co-script.
L'homme en colère (Claude Pinoteau). Co-script.
Ils sont grands, ces petits (Joël Santoni). Co-adaptation.
Retour à la bien-aimée (Jean-François Adam). Co-script.
L'associé (René Gainville). Co-script.

1980 *Sauve qui peut (la vie) / Every Man for Himself* (Jean-Luc Godard). Co-script.

1981 *Black Mirror* (Pierre-Alain Jollivet). Co-script.
Die Fälschung / Circle of Deceit (Volker Schlöndorff). Co-script.

1982 *Le retour de Martin Guerre / The Return of Martin Guerre* (Daniel Vigne). Co-script.
Passion (Jean-Luc Godard). Uncredited contribution.
L'indiscrétion (Pierre Lary). Co-script.
Antonieta (Carlos Saura). Story, co-script.

1983 *Danton* (Andrzej Wajda). Co-script.
Itinéraire bis (Christian Drillaud). Co-script.
Il generale dell'armata morte (Luciano Tovoli). Co-script.
La tragédie de Carmen (Peter Brook). Co-adaptation.

1984 *Un amour de Swann / Swann in Love* (Volker Schlöndorff). Co-script.

1985 *Auto défense* (Hervé Lavayssière). Script (short film).

1986 *L'unique* (Jean-Claude Carrière and Jérôme Diamant-Berger). Co-director, co-script.
La joven y la tentación (François Mimet). Script.
Max mon amour (Nagashi Oshima). Idea and co-scenario.
Oviri (Henning Carlsen). Co-scenario.
La dernière image (Mohammad Lakhdar-Hamina). Co-adaptation.

1987 *Les exploits d'un jeune Don Juan* (Gianfranco Mingozzi). Co-script.

1988 *The Unbearable Lightness of Being* (Philip Kaufman). Co-script.
Les possédés (Andrzej Wajda). Dialogue and scenario.
La nuit bengali (Nicolas Klotz). Script.
Max mon amour (Nagisa Oshima). Idea and co-scenario.
1989 *Valmont* (Milos Forman). Co-script.
J'écris dans l'espace (Pierre Etaix). Co-script.
1990 *Milou en mai / May Fools* (Louis Malle). Co-script.
Es ist nicht leicht ein Gott zu sein (Peter Fleischmann). Co-script.
Cyrano de Bergerac (Jean-Paul Rappenau). Co-script.
1991 *At Play in the Fields of the Lord* (Hector Babenco). Co-script.
1992 *Le retour de Casanova* (Edouard Niemans). Script.
1993 *Sommersby* (Jon Amiel). American remake of *The Return of Martin Guerre.*
1995 *The Night and the Moment* (Anna Maria Tatò). Co-script.
Le hussard sur le toit (Jean-Paul Rappenau). Co-script.
1996 *Der Unhold / The Ogre* (Volker Schlöndorff). Co-script.
Golden Boy (Jean-Pierre Vergne). Co-script.
The Associate (Donald Petrie). American remake of *L'associé.*
1997 *Les paradoxes de Buñuel* (Jorge Amat). Co-script (documentary).
Chinese Box (Wayne Wang). Co-story, co-script.
1998 *Attaville, la véritable histoire des fourmis* (Gérald Calderon). Commentary (documentary).
1999 *Broken Dolls* (Jesus Franco). Uncredited contribution.
La guerre dans le Haut Pays (Francis Reusser). Co-script.
2000 *Salsa* (Joyce Buñuel). Co-script.
2003 *Rien, voilà l'ordre* (Jacques Baratier). Co-script.
2004 *Birth* (Jonathan Glazer). Co-script.
2006 *Goya's Ghosts* (Milos Forman). Co-script.
2007 *Ulzhan* (Volker Schlöndorff). Co-script.

Television includes *La reine verte* (1964); *Les aventures de Robinson Crusoë* (multiple episodes, 1964); *Le franc-tireur* (1978); *Photo-souvenir* (1978); *Harold et Maud* (French adaptation, 1978); *Mesure pour mesure* (French adaptation, 1979); *Lundi* (1980); *Le bouffon* (1981); *La double vie de Théophraste Longuet* (1981); *Je tue il* (1982); *La cerisaie* (1982); *L'accompagnateur* (1982); *Les secrets de la princesse de Cadignan* (1982);

Credo (1983); *Le jardinier récalcitrant* (1983); *L'aide-mémoire* (1984); *Les étonnements d'un couple moderne* (1985); *Bouvard et Pecuchet* (1989); *Une femme tranquille* (1989); *L'héritage de la chouette* (miniseries, 1989); *The Mahabharata* (miniseries, 1989); *La controverse de Valladolid* (1992); *Associations de bienfaiteurs* (miniseries, 1995); *La Duchesse de Langeais* (1995); *Le parfum de Jeannette* (1996); *Une femme explosive* (1996); *Clarissa* (1998); *Bérénice* (2000); *Lettre d'une inconnue* (French adaptation, 2001); *Madame de . . .* (French adaptation, 2001); *La bataille d'Hernani* (2002); *Ruy Blas* (2002); *Les Thibault* (miniseries, 2003); *Le père Goriot* (2004); *Galilée, ou L'amour de Dieu* (2005); *Marie-Antoinette* (2006); *Le rêve* (series, 2006).

Published plays include (partial listing for English-language books only) *The Little Black Book, The Conference of the Birds, The Mahabharata,* and *The Controversy of Valladolid.*

Other published works include (partial listing for English-language books only) *Monsieur Hulot's Holiday* (novelization); *May Fools* (published screenplay); *The Secret Language of Film* (nonfiction); *Violence and Compassion* (with the Dalai Lama); *In Search of the Mahabharata;* and *Please, Mr. Einstein.*

Academy Award honors include an Oscar in 1963, shared with Pierre Etaix for Best Short Subject, Live Action, for *Heureux anniversaire;* a nomination in 1973 for Best Screenplay Based on Material Not Previously Published or Produced, for *The Discreet Charm of the Bourgeoisie* (shared with Luis Buñuel); a nomination in 1978 for Best Screenplay Based on Material from Another Medium, for *That Obscure Object of Desire* (shared with Buñuel); and a nomination in 1989 for Best Screenplay Based on Material from Another Medium in 1989, for *The Unbearable Lightness of Being* (shared with Philip Kaufman).

Writers Guild of America honors include the Laurel Award for lifetime screenwriting achievement in 2000. Carrière was nominated in 1972 for Best Original Comedy script for *Taking Off* (shared with Milos Forman, John Guare, and Jon Klein), and nominated in 1989 for Best Adapted Script for *The Unbearable Lightness of Being* (shared with Philip Kaufman).

INTERVIEW BY **PATRICK McGILLIGAN**

NORA EPHRON FEMINIST WITH A FUNNY BONE

Nora Ephron has several careers, which she has shuffled like a master dealer always with one more card up her sleeve.

Long before her first screen credit, she was well known as one of the leading voices of New Journalism, a tough reporter, first-person essayist, and feminist with a funny bone—sometimes one or the other, other times all three at once. Three collections of her newspaper and magazine pieces became best-selling books in the 1970s. Her first marriage was to writer Dan Greenburg; her second was newsworthy: Carl Bernstein, one of the two *Washington Post* reporters who pushed the Watergate story until Nixon resigned. (The disintegration of their marriage was channeled into Ephron's first novel, *Heartburn,* later filmed by Mike Nichols from a script by Ephron.) High on the Who's Who of East Coast literary lights, she even appeared as a party guest in two Woody Allen films.

When she turned to scriptwriting in the early 1980s, Ephron was, in a sense, coming home to Hollywood. Her personal backstory included a childhood growing up in Los Angeles, as the oldest of four daughters of Henry and Phoebe Ephron, who together wrote plays like *Take Her She's Mine* and a number of sparkling motion pictures, including *There's No Business Like Show Business* (1954), the screen version of *Carousel* (1956), and the Hepburn-Tracy comedy *Desk Set* (1957), capping their scriptwriting careers with an Oscar nomination for adapting *Captain Newman, M.D.* in 1964. *We Thought We Could Do Anything: The Life of Screenwriters Phoebe and Henry Ephron* (1977) is Henry Ephron's elegant memoir of the family's life out west, with a moving introduction by Nora and many glimpses of her precocity as a child. Her parents were displaced New Yorkers, and she did not much like California (or Hollywood). After education at Wellesley she ended up in New York working for newspapers, which she highly recommends for budding scenarists looking for better training than film school.

After dipping her toes in television in the late 1970s, she was asked by director Mike Nichols to write a true-life script about the suspicious car-crash death of antinuclear crusader and union activist Karen Silkwood. The gritty, disturbing *Silkwood,* which starred Meryl Streep (who later played the Ephron character in the film *Heartburn*), brought Ephron her first Oscar nomination in 1983. *Silkwood* performed only modestly at the box office compared to the hilarious romantic comedy *When Harry Met Sally,* which was a runaway crowd-pleaser in 1989, swiftly achieving iconic status among writers as well as fans, for its smart script probing the limits of platonic friendship between a man (Harry, played by Billy Crystal) and a woman (Sally, played by Meg Ryan) who are sexually attracted to each other. (Everyone knows the scene in crowded Katz's Deli, where Harry is insisting he can't be fooled by a woman's pretend orgasm. Sally, loudly and vividly, fakes one to win the argument, topped by—it was Billy Crystal's suggestion, which Ephron added to the script—a woman customer shouting out, "I'll have what she's having!") Ephron collected a second Oscar nomination for this film.

She crashed the boy's club of directing in 1992 with *This Is My Life,* based on a Meg Wolitzer novel about a single mother finding a second chance in stand-up comedy. Then she was called in on an informal remake of Leo McCarey's *An Affair to Remember* (1957), and her witty final script (again, Oscar nominated) and growingly assured direction transformed *Sleepless in Seattle* into the perfect date movie of 1993.

During the 1980s, Alice Arlen was her regular collaborator; on more recent projects younger sister Delia has served in that capacity. Things came full circle in 1998 when Ephron reunited *Sleepless in Seattle* stars Tom Hanks and Meg Ryan in *You've Got Mail,* the Ephron sisters' Internet-themed update of Ernst Lubitsch's *The Shop around the Corner* (1940); one of their parents' earliest jobs in Hollywood had been on the last Lubitsch film (*That Lady in Ermine,* 1948) before the master of sophisticated comedy died.

Along the way there has been a kooky-teenager-with-mobster-dad drama (*Cookie,* 1989); the underrated *My Blue Heaven* (1990) and *Mixed Nuts* (1994), both starring Steve Martin; *Michael* (1996), which features John Travolta as an angel luring all the women out on the floor of a roadhouse for a magical dance to "Chain of Fools"; *Hanging Up* (2000), an adaptation with Delia of her sister's novel for the actress—and in this instance, director—Diane Keaton; another Travolta vehicle, *Lucky Numbers*

(2000), which is the only time Ephron has directed a film from someone else's script; and the big-screen version of TV's *Bewitched* (2005), with Nicole Kidman and Will Ferrell, which inexplicably fizzled.

Her comedies embrace the McCarey-Lubitsch tradition, albeit with a hip female sensibility. Her journalistic dramas have proven harder to sell to an increasingly homogenized Hollywood. Lately she's shifted her energies into a play (*Imaginary Friends,* about the relationship, anything but friendly, between novelist-essayist Mary McCarthy and playwright Lillian Hellman), and to fresh journalism (leading to another best-selling book, *I Feel Bad about My Neck: And Other Thoughts on Being a Woman,* in 2006). She still prefers New York, where she lives with her husband, crime writer Nicholas Pileggi, who is also an occasional screenwriter (*Goodfellas*).

In the spirit of *You've Got Mail* this interview was conducted by e-mail.

• • •

You once said that a helpful strategy for you as a journalist was to write as though you were writing a letter to your mother and then lop off the salutation. I have a feeling that strategy doesn't work as well for film, even though your mother—and father—were scriptwriters. Who is your imagined ideal reader for any script that you are writing? (And is it the same as your imagined ideal audience for the film?)

Actually, I didn't exactly say that. (Although who knows?) What I hope I said is that my mother used to quote George Bernard Shaw, who may or may not have said, the best way to learn to write is to write a letter to your mother and cut off the "Dear Mom." Just quoting that makes me know absolutely that George Bernard Shaw never said anything of the kind. But my mother definitely did, and definitely attributed it to someone. No question it was very helpful to me in becoming a journalist, in that becoming comfortable with your voice is part of what makes it possible to write a column, make a joke in print, etc.

I don't think it works at all in screenwriting, though. But I suspect I've always had ideal readers for my scripts, though different ideal readers for each one. (The same was true when I became a columnist and magazine writer, I always had an ideal reader.)

No question that my ideal reader for screenplays was often Mike Nichols, because I learned so much about screenwriting from him. And occasionally (in the case of *You've Got Mail*) the ideal reader was Tom Hanks, because I hoped he would play the lead, and because I learned so much about screenwriting from him. When I wrote *When Harry Met*

Sally, I was writing it for Rob Reiner, whose idea it was—so he was my ideal reader.

Although you are a "child of Hollywood," you spent years in journalism and a long time doing other things before coming around to film. There aren't many "children of Hollywood" who are second- or third-generation screenwriters. It's as though, early on, you (and they) had become hyper-aware of the pitfalls. In your case, what took you so long? I have a suspicion it wasn't merely happenstance.

Well, I never wanted to be in the movie business when I was growing up. For one thing, it would have meant living in Los Angeles. No one in the movie business in the 1950s lived anywhere else. I would have died if I'd had to live in Los Angeles. From the moment we moved there for good, in 1946, when I was five, I knew a terrible mistake had been made. For another thing, the movie business was clearly not a good business for women. And for a third thing, I didn't want to be in the movie business, I wanted to be a journalist. It was only after I'd been a journalist for years that I tried screenwriting. By then, you could live in New York and be in the movie business, thank God.

In what I like to refer to as the "so-called golden age" of Hollywood, many scriptwriters honed their writing skills on newspapers and magazines. Today Hollywood is flooded with film (and business) school graduates. Few screenwriters come from journalism. Journalism itself isn't what it used to be, but it's like Hollywood has dropped it as part of the curriculum. And I feel that not only are their fewer "journalistic" movies, but that the lack of scriptwriters with newspaper background contributes to the homogenization of scripts and films. Do you agree? What is the most important thing you learned as a journalist, that helps with every script?

I always tell kids who want to go to film school that they should become journalists instead. And I always tell journalists they should write screenplays. But no one listens to me. What I loved about journalism is that you learn a great deal about all the things you write about; in my case I was very lucky, and wrote about pretty much everything: crimes, politics, fluff, famous people, New York, heat waves, real estate, the women's movement, journalism, to name a few. Then, if you want to write screenplays, you at least know something about something.

When Alice Arlen and I wrote *Silkwood*, I knew all sorts of things—how to report a story, most importantly. But I also knew about unions because I'd been active in the Newspaper Guild at the *New York Post.* And I knew what people talked about at work. And I also understood structure in an instinctive way, because one of the things you learn as a magazine journalist is Beginning, Middle, End, which is pretty much the main thing you have to understand when you write a screenplay.

There are still numerous "films based on true-life events," but not many feel true-to-life and there are often sentimental script contrivances. Films like Silkwood, *in which you honestly "report a story," are few and far between (if not virtually extinct in Hollywood) nowadays. What is the special responsibility of such a script, based on actual characters and events?*

My feeling is that these scripts have a real responsibility to—well, not to facts, because there are very few real "facts"—but to certain things that you simply can't change because (as Richard Nixon once put it) it would be wrong.

You can't write *Silkwood* and make Karen Silkwood into a saint. She wasn't a saint. One of the things that was hard for me at the beginning with *Silkwood,* by the way, was that most of the journalism that had been written about her had been one-sided, either painting her as a saint or as a hysteric. When Alice Arlen and I interviewed Karen's boyfriend Drew Stevens, he told us that she had flashed her breasts one day in the plutonium plant, and I suddenly understood her. Having Meryl Streep involved with the project from the beginning was also very helpful, because we knew that she would be able to play a complicated young woman and so we were going to be free to write one.

Anyway, my feeling is that when you write a story that's based on actual characters and events, there are certain marks you have to hit, that you have an obligation to, even as a screenwriter. So in the case of Karen Silkwood, you had to make her complicated, you had to make her difficult, and obviously there were certain factual moments that you absolutely had to include. But there's no rule; you sort of know what they are. On the other hand, Alice and I seriously fiddled with the length of time involved. The movie takes events that took place over a couple of years and makes them into a much shorter time period. Alice is brilliant at structure, among other things, and this was very much her idea.

You say that you preferred journalism, early on, and at first had no intentions of writing films. I know you did some interesting television, starting out, but what is it exactly (or as exactly as you might be able to say) that ultimately made you turn to scriptwriting?

I didn't do any interesting television. I did a script for a women's caper movie that sold to television. It was the first thing I did that was produced, and it wasn't good.

What mostly made me turn to screenwriting is that everyone in New York was sort of trying to get into screenwriting. Carl Bernstein and I had done some work on the script of *All the President's Men* (1976) in a misguided attempt to convey to Alan Pakula and Robert Redford some of the things that he and Bob Woodward felt were missing from the original draft. Someone saw the work I'd done and suggested I write a women's caper movie, which I did. And it sold to television. As I said, it wasn't a good movie but it wasn't a bad script, so I started to get work as a screenwriter. Which was lucky.

Can you characterize what Mike Nichols taught you?

He taught me many many things. Here are two: (1) To look at each scene of the movie and say, "What is this section of the movie called?" And whatever the answer is, that's what the scene has to be about. And if six scenes in a row are all called the same thing, then you'd better fix that because you have too many scenes that are all about the same thing. (2) To free-associate whenever you work on a scene. So if the scene is about a breakup, you should basically thinks about all the breakups you've known. The same goes for falling in love, or betrayal, or whatever. It's a way of using psychoanalysis and writing together, and it is, of course, the reason why Mike Nichols's breakup with one of his girlfriends ended up in *Silkwood.*

Why, after Silkwood *(and, to an extent,* Heartburn*), does it seem, at least judging from your official credits, that you left "reportorial" and "journalistic" films behind? Is that to some extent because of Hollywood and what the market will bear? Changing times, happenstance? Or did you write other hard-hitting, true-story scripts that weren't filmed?*

I have written two scripts that are reportorial. One about Maggie Higgins, who won a Pulitzer Prize for covering the Korean War for the *New York Herald-Tribune.* Alice Arlen and I wrote it together, and it is one of the heartbreaks of my life as a screenwriter that it was never made. It came this close several times. The other is called "Stories about McAlary," about a man named Mike McAlary who also won a Pulitzer, writing for the *Daily News.* I hope that Home Box Office is going to make it.

It also seems that with When Harry Met Sally *you came "home" to a strong suit that had been waiting for you to take it up. To some extent, "home" to the tradition of your parents (with films like* Desk Set*) and the evergreen tradition of romantic comedy. Can you talk about how and why you got the job, and how the project started out, versus how it ended up?*

The idea for it was Rob Reiner's: let's do a movie about two people who become friends at the end of the first major relationships of their lives, and make a decision not to have sex because it ruins the relationship, and then they have sex and it ruins the relationship. That's where it began. I interviewed Rob and Andy Scheinman (the producer) about their lives as single men, and basically approached the script as an essay on being single. Then, around the third draft or so, they interviewed me, and that's where the orgasm scene began. There is quite a long description of the whole thing in the introduction to the published screenplay of *When Harry Met Sally.*[1]

The orgasm scene was of course started by Rob and Andy and me, made into a legend by Meg Ryan (whose idea it was for Sally to have the orgasm at the end of the scene), and by Billy Crystal (who thought of the line "I'll have what she's having"). I learned in the course of that movie that if an actor wants to change something for the better, you would have to be a fool to object.

Are you conscious, having at one time described yourself as a radical feminist (I'm sure you're the same now, only different), of always struggling with the clichés of romantic comedy? After all, you once wrote, "So many of the conscious and unconscious ways men and women treat each other have to do with romantic and sexual fantasies that are deeply ingrained, not just in society but in literature." And of course Hollywood plays a big part!

When did I describe myself as a radical feminist? I'm a feminist but never a radical feminist to the best of my memory. But yes, I still agree with that quote. And of course Hollywood plays a big part. That's one of the subjects in all my romantic comedies—the role of other movies (or, in the case of *You've Got Mail,* books) in that fantasy.

It's interesting when you talk about the contribution of Billy Crystal to When Harry Met Sally. *I can't help but notice you are fond of casting other actors who were once stand-up comedians and who might be counted on to be freewheeling with their ideas and performances: Steve Martin, Dan Aykroyd, Tom Hanks, even Will Farrell. Do your comedy scripts in particular remain fluid for the actors?*

Tom Hanks was never a stand-up comedian, and Rob Reiner cast Billy Crystal in *When Harry Met Sally*. But many actors who are funny began as stand-up comedians, so you inevitably (when casting someone funny) are going to cast people who began as stand-up comedians. I learned on *When Harry Met Sally* that you have to remain open to change, especially when you're directing comedy. What's the point of casting all these people who are comedically gifted if you don't take advantage of their brilliance at comedy and improvisation?

When I started out as a screenwriter, everyone knew about the legendary screenwriter Paddy Chayefsky, whose contract stipulated that you could not change one word of his screenplay. Everyone thought this was a goal worth having, contract-wise. But after I worked with Rob and Billy and Meg on *When Harry Met Sally*, it crossed my mind that Chayevsky had no understanding at all of the movie-making process.

Every time I quote something you said in the past I seem to get it a little wrong, but in one of your long-ago profiles you wrote about a pioneering lady umpire (I think) and the "ridicule and abuse" women must undergo when they pioneer in a male-dominated profession. I can't think of a more male-dominated profession than directing motion pictures, still. Why did you take up that job?

Well, being the first woman umpire is very different from being a director, and I was hardly the first woman director. The hardest thing about being a woman director is not the directing part—if you have a crew that's good and you are careful not to hire Australian cameramen and you're prepared, you'll be fine. But the hard part is getting movies made that are not slam-dunk action pictures, which most women don't direct and (in my case) aren't interested in directing.

You said you "learned" a lot about screenwriting from Tom Hanks during Sleepless in Seattle. *Can you tell me more about that? And at what stage did you take over the script and directing?*

I came onto *Sleepless* to do a three-week polish for a director who was already attached to a go-picture with actors who were semi-cast. At least three writers had been on the project before me. The script I polished was not a comedy, it was sort of gloopy, but it had all sorts of things about it that worked, particularly the ending at the Empire State Building. I made it funny and basically made the woman's part better and the kid's part better. When I turned it in, there was a sort of feeding frenzy for the script—a huge number of actors wanted to be in it. Everyone loved it. I've never had anything quite like it happen. Everyone loved it except for the director who was attached, so he withdrew.

So the people at Tri-Star asked me if I wanted to direct it, and long story short, I said yes. As for the actors—the actress also withdrew, perhaps understanding that she was not funny, which she isn't; and the actor, who hadn't made a deal to be in the movie, was just shunted aside in favor of Tom. But Tom felt that his part was underwritten—which it was, by the way, and he didn't commit until he and I and Delia had spent quite a lot of time together going scene by scene through the script. During which meetings, Tom would say, "Well I wouldn't exactly say this"—and then he'd improvise what he would say, and it was brilliant and funny and we would write it down and basically put it into the script. All sorts of great things in the script of *Sleepless* came from Tom's mouth in those meetings, including much of the best part of his phone call with Dr. Marsha, the radio talk-show host. But what I learned from Tom was a thing that's really important, which is that scene after scene, you have to give the main actor something to play, he can never be passive in the scene, et cetera, even (or especially) when he's sharing it with a very cute little boy.

Can you talk a little about collaborating on scripts with your sister Delia? The fun or unique chemistry of it? I can't think of too many other female-sibling partnerships nowadays. It's almost like channeling your parents!

I love working with Delia because she makes me laugh more than anyone I know. I started working with her on the first movie I directed—*This Is My Life.* I had by then deluded myself into thinking that I had been wildly helpful to the directors I'd worked with as a screenwriter, and in any case, I wanted to make sure someone was there playing that role for me when I started directing. I knew for sure, in addition, that I'd need someone to make changes and have a cold clear eye out for the script. When you start directing, you really aren't looking out for the script—you're elsewhere. Anyway, it turned out to be exactly what I'd hoped for, and a chance for me to spend way more time than I normally would with one of my favorite people.

June 2007

NORA EPHRON (1941–)

1983 *Silkwood* (Mike Nichols). Co-script.

1986 *Heartburn* (Mike Nichols). Script (based on her novel).

1989 *When Harry Met Sally* (Rob Reiner). Associate producer, script.
Cookie (Susan Seidelman). Executive producer, co-script.
1990 *My Blue Heaven* (Herbert Ross). Executive producer, script.
1992 *This Is My Life* (Nora Ephron). Director, co-script.
1993 *Sleepless in Seattle* (Nora Ephron). Director, co-script.
1994 *Mixed Nuts* (Nora Ephron). Director, co-script.
1996 *Michael* (Nora Ephron). Producer, director, co-script.
1998 *You've Got Mail* (Nora Ephron). Producer, director, co-script.
Strike! / aka *All I Wanna Do* (Sarah Kernochan). Executive producer.
2000 *Hanging Up* (Diane Keaton). Producer, co-script (based on Delia Ephron's novel).
Lucky Numbers (Nora Ephron). Producer, director.
2005 *Bewitched* (Nora Ephron). Producer, director, co-script.
2008 *Flipped* (Nora Ephron). Director, co-script.
2009 *Julie and Julia* (Nora Ephron). Director, script.

Television includes *Adam's Rib* (1973 series) and *Perfect Gentleman* (writer of 1978 telefilm).

Academy Award honors include a Best Original Screenplay nomination in 1984, for *Silkwood* (shared with Alice Arlen); a Best Original Screenplay nomination in 1990, for *When Harry Met Sally;* and a Best Original Screenplay nomination in 1994, for *Sleepless in Seattle* (shared with David S. Ward and Jeff Arch).

Writers Guild honors include earning the 2003 Ian McLellan Hunter Award for lifetime screenwriting achievement. The Writers Guild has nominated Ephron three times for Best Original Screenplay: for *Silkwood, When Harry Met Sally,* and *Sleepless in Seattle.*

NOTE

1 The *When Harry Met Sally* screenplay was published as a paperback by Knopf in 1990.

INTERVIEW BY **PATRICK McGILLIGAN**

RONALD HARWOOD IMAGINATION

Ronald Harwood speaks of the theater as his "natural habitat," as is only fitting for a man who has written three dozen noteworthy plays, nonfiction books, and histories of the stage. His name is synonymous with quality theater in England, and his life's work has led to him being made a Commander of the British Empire (CBE), among many other high recognitions.

At the same time, dating back forty-five years to his early brushes with film—particularly his first major credit on Alexander Mackendrick's film of Richard Hughes's novel *A High Wind in Jamaica* (1965)—he has been nearly as prolific and accomplished at his sideline of writing motion pictures, becoming over the years a stealth candidate for the master adapter of the profession.

Sometimes the films are tricky adaptations of his own plays, other times they are trickier adaptations of beloved novels by world-famous authors as diverse as Alexander Solzhenitsyn, Alan Paton, Charles Dickens, Somerset Maugham, and Gabriel García Márquez. As this list suggests, Harwood, a Londoner by way of South Africa and a onetime president of International PEN, has been the most worldly of screenwriters, writing acclaimed films that are presented in foreign languages and for directors as diverse as the Finnish-born Caspar Wrede, the Hungarian Istvan Szabo, and the displaced Parisian Roman Polanski. Harwood has been nominated for an Oscar three times, and won, in 2002, for his script of *The Pianist,* directed by Polanski, based on the memoir by Wladyslaw Szpilman about his struggle for survival in wartime Warsaw.

Harwood has been peaking as a screenwriter for the last ten years, seeming to specialize in bravura projects that would daunt, or at least slow down, a lesser mortal. The year 2007 was especially remarkable, with his adaptations of the Gabriel García Márquez novel *Love in the Time of Cholera* for the English director Mike Newell, and the Jean-Dominique Bauby memoir *The Diving Bell and the Butterfly* for the American Julian Schnabel. (The script for *The Diving Bell and the Butterfly* may have lost the Oscar to the Coen brothers in Hollywood, but Harwood's adaptation won the top prize in its category at the British Academy of Film and Television Arts awards.) Two more disparate or difficult adaptations it would be hard to imagine, but a Ronald Harwood script has become a guarantee of excellence.

. . .

Growing up in South Africa as you did, I gather you fell in love with theater. But were you following films at all? British and Australian only, or Hollywood as well? With any idea that films too had scripts and writers. . . ?

I saw British and Hollywood films. I don't think I ever saw an Australian film. (Were there any?) The first film I saw, aged six, was *The Mark of Zorro* (1940) with Tyrone Power. When I was a little older we used to go to the cinema (in those days called the "bioscope" by South Africans) on Saturday mornings and see serials and comedy shorts.

It never occurred to me that films had scripts. I think the first time I had any notion of a screenplay was when I saw Olivier's *Hamlet* (1948) and *Henry V* (1944), because I realized that Shakespeare had to be adapted for the screen. Alan Dent was credited as "script advisor" and I knew his name because he was a well-known London theater critic. But I don't think I showed any interest in other screenwriters until I saw *The Third Man* in 1949 or 1950, and that was because I knew and was greatly influenced by the novels of Graham Greene. I was impressed that so famous a writer also wrote for the screen.

What is the first thing you wrote (article, poem, script, or whatever) for which you were paid actual money?

A novel, called in England *All the Same Shadows* and in the USA, *George Washington September, Sir!*

When you were serving as "the dresser," did you know instinctively that one day you were going to write it all up? And were you taking notes or relying on memory?

No, not at all. I had no idea I would be a writer when I was Sir Donald Wolfit's dresser. My burning ambition was to be an actor. And I never make notes, not then, not now. I have a theory that ideas or events, if important, will be remembered.

What—and why—was your first professional involvement with film?

A short feature film (just over an hour in length) was made of my first television play, *The Barber of Stamford Hill* (1962). The play had been very well received in 1960 when it was first shown. Two years later, the director Casper Wrede and I were approached by a young producer, Ben Arbeid, who somehow managed to finance the movie. It was made at Shepperton Studios. The first day of filming was the first time I'd ever visited a film studio.

Casper Wrede is not a well-known name on this side of the Atlantic, yet you appear to have had a long, fond, productive relationship with him, right through to your Solzhenitsyn adaptation. Starting out, how did he help or complement you as a screenwriter, or were you learning the ropes of film together?

He was a very important figure in my life. Finnish-born of an aristocratic family—he was a baron—he came to England in the early 1950s to study theater directing at the Old Vic School. In 1959 he was one of the founders of the 59 Theatre Company at the Lyric Theatre, Hammersmith. My wife, Natasha, was employed as their stage manager and, through her, I was employed as a small-part actor. I sent him my first TV play, *The Barber of Stamford Hill,* which he liked and directed. We then made the film and later another film of my second TV play, *Private Potter* (1962), with Tom Courtenay. We were learning the ropes together, as you say.

One Day in the Life of Ivan Denisovich is a film of which I am very proud. Casper directed it wonderfully and Sven Nykvist shot it magnificently. Tom Courtenay was pretty good, too.

A High Wind in Jamaica *was one of the first "serious" films I ever saw, I think because my mother took us, thinking it was a "family movie" because it had a cast of children. At least three writers are credited in most sources. Is there any way to sort out your individual contribution, or what you brought to the film script?*

I couldn't possibly be accurate about it now. [Director Alexander] Mackendrick told me that most of it was mine but dialogue was added by the others. He may just have said that to reassure or flatter me.

The novel of A High Wind in Jamaica *is so concise, so compressed, and some key aspects are changed in the film, but what really impressed me (viewing the film again and rereading the book) is how the Anthony Quinn character and the girl Emily bring the audience into the story; the sharpening of their characterizations and their relationship give the film its point of view. Obviously you were feeling free to depart and invent, while writing the script. Does that have more to do with the shortish, elliptical nature of the novel? Mackendrick's approach? Or your own instincts?*

I suppose I don't dare add the question, "What did you teach Martin Amis about writing while he was flirting with acting?"[1]

It is such a long time ago that I find it difficult to remember the process. I suspect that the approach belonged more to Mackendrick than to me. All I do know is he taught me a tremendous amount about construction and the screenplay form. He was a superb teacher.

On the rare occasions I see Martin Amis I always say to him, "If you'd only stuck to acting I could have made you a star."

I know it's unfair to ask you everything that Mackendrick taught you about screenplay structure and form. But, in an anecdote or as an example, can you give me a taste of what he taught you?

He taught me about designing sequences using postcards. You wrote each scene on a card, laid them out on a board or on the floor, and shuffled them around until you were more or less happy with the result.

Something else he taught me was to be as economical as possible when describing a setting or an action.

My first stab at the screenplay—for Sandy's eyes only—began, as the novel begins, with a two or three page description of the wind starting to rise, using much of Hughes's descriptive language from the book. Sandy looked at it, noisily cleared his nose or throat, and asked, "What's this?"

"The sea becoming rough and the wind beginning to rise," I said. "From the book."

"Cut it," he said. "Put what you've just said: 'The sea becomes rough and the wind rises.' I'll do the rest." It was my first lesson in keeping description to a minimum and to avoid literary pretensions in a screenplay.

I'm guessing that most of your film work during the 1960s was, to one extent or another, serendipity, or jobs of work. More than once there are multiple writers. Some of those films are hard to hunt up on video or DVD over here in America. Both Drop Dead Darling *and* Diamonds for Breakfast *sound like fun.* Eyewitness *is the intriguing one; John Hough was sometimes an exceptional director in this period, though he never quite broke out of the pack. Do you take special pride or responsibility in any one of these films, more than the others?*

I was trying to make a living. I used (or misused) movies to finance my novels and plays. [Director] Ken Hughes employed me fairly frequently but would never let me share the screenplay credit. All I remember of John Hough is him throwing up in my car after lunch.

I also worked for Italian directors during that period. They had screenplays literally translated from Italian into English. They wanted someone to make the English version readable. I had a wonderful time being flown back and forth to Rome, first class, and put up in splendid hotels. I worked with Valerio Zurlini, Mario Monicelli, and a fine screenwriter, Suso Cecci-d'Amico. The only screenplay of the ones I worked on that was made into a film (mostly in London) was *La ragazza con la pistola* ("The Girl with a Gun," 1968) starring Monica Vitti.

The important thing to me about that period was that, unknowingly, I was being well paid to learn my craft.

I heard an excellent interview with you on National Public Radio here in America about Love in the Time of Cholera, *in which you said you had never met Gabriel García Márquez, and it was my impression that you said this almost as a matter of policy. Did you meet or consult with Solzhenitsyn when doing* One Day in the Life of Ivan Denisovich? *Is it policy, when you are adapting someone else's work, or does it depend on the project?*

It is a matter of policy. And no, I didn't meet Solzhenitsyn because he was in the Soviet Union and exiled at about the time the film was finished. I am always concerned that the source author will insist that some incident or sequence in the book or play is essential to the movie, when you know very well it has no place in the film at all. It is difficult enough adapting a work to the screen without unnecessary inhibitions imposed by the original author.

I gather that when your play The Dresser *was filmed in 1983, your collaboration with the director was especially close and that you exerted an unusual degree of influence over the production. I believe it is the only time you have taken a "producer" credit. (I'm surprised you weren't tempted to direct.) Were there any major changes from the play, and what were the key things you did behind the scenes that you don't do on your typical job for hire?*

All due to the generosity and decency of Peter Yates. I did not "take" a producer credit. Peter gave it to me. He drove my wife and me up Sunset

Boulevard to Westwood to show me a huge ad on the corner of a building which had his and my name above the title. I can't remember whether or not I was listed as a producer on the actual film credits.

The main change is what some people call "opening out" but I like to call "opening in," trying to extract scenes spoken about IN the play, and then dramatizing them, for example, the market scene and Sir's breakdown. But most importantly is the railway station scene ("STOP THAT TRAIN!") which Norman, the dresser, talks about in the play. I added the train stopping, which was an apocryphal story about Wolfit that I'd heard when I was working for him. It was telling Peter Yates this story when we first met that convinced him we could make a film of the subject.

About The Doctor and the Devils: *the Dylan Thomas script had been kicking around for over three decades. What were its big problems, and what did you do to solve them?*

I don't like talking about this film. I don't think I did a good job and I certainly didn't solve the problems, which all stemmed from Dylan Thomas's amazing and bewitching use of language.

I assume the policy of avoiding the original author goes out the window when we are talking about the subject of a film, rather than the source material. But perhaps I am wrong. Did you spend much time with Nelson Mandela when writing your script about him? It must have been a privilege—and responsibility—to write about such a great man. Can you tell me how you approached the facts in terms of organizing the drama? Do you always do some research?

Nelson Mandela was in prison when I wrote the screenplay. It's a long time ago now and I cannot remember the details of my research. There was much written material available. I talked to several people who knew him, mostly ANC people in exile, but they all were too reverential to be trusted.

I am always careful not to attribute to real people views they do not hold, or that there is no proof for them holding.

Of course, I always do some research, especially if one is dealing with historical characters and times.

Cry, the Beloved Country *must also have been a privilege and responsibility. I feel certain you must have read the book when you were young, and that you were trying to be faithful to an old friend, the book. Am I wrong? Does one's personal attachment to a story (as opposed, say, to purely professional respect or admiration) make a difference in one's willingness to depart from it? I'm guessing you approached* Oliver Twist *with the same fondness.*

Yes, *Cry the Beloved Country* was the first book I read, in adolescence, which opened my eyes to apartheid.

No, I don't think my personal attachment to the book had any influence on my adaptation. All one wants to do is adapt the book to the best of one's ability. Same is true of *Oliver Twist,* from which I cut the entire subplot.

Dickens is such a great storyteller that it is best to follow the events as he tells them with whatever cuts are deemed necessary to bring the story down to a manageable cinematic length. I did not try to bypass Fagin being a Jew. In my first draft, however, I did not include the scene with Fagin and Oliver in the condemned cell. Roman insisted it go in. I went back to my Paris flat that evening and worked into the early hours, hammering out the scene. I read it to Polanski the next morning (for some reason he likes me to read the script to him), and he said, "That's great, really great," and it was shot as written.

Do you feel more of an obligation to hew to a play and playwright? I'm thinking of Terence Rattigan *and* The Browning Version. *After all, plays are already well known for a certain sequence of scenes and precise dialogue, and that is what sophisticated theater audiences will expect from a film version. Whereas books as a rule open themselves up to more freedom . . . don't they?*

Plays, for me, are more difficult to adapt precisely because there are inevitably long dialogue scenes, often in one location. Plays are about language, cinema about visual images. So one has to translate the language of the play into the visual demands of the cinema.

How about in terms of your own plays that are filmed? What were the changes you made in turning your play about Wilhelm Furtwängler into the film Taking Sides, *for Istvan Szabo?*[2] *Major or minor changes? Szabo's films are rarely shown over here, and just as rare in DVD.*

As far as my own plays go, my rule is to abandon the play as far as possible and reinvent for the cinema. I look at what is spoken about in the play and see if these references can be developed into scenes and sequences, as I've already mentioned in regard to *The Dresser.*

Most of the changes in *Taking Sides* were made by me. Szabo made many suggestions which I incorporated. I think that when he saw I was able to cut myself free from the rigid demands of the play, he felt free to suggest, invent, and insist. It was a very happy relationship.

How did you get connected with The Pianist? *Did you have some background with Roman Polanski?*

I met Polanski once in Moscow in the 1980s when we were both there to doing some research on separate projects. We met at breakfast and he told me he was a fan of *The Dresser.* Then, my play *Taking Sides* was running in Paris in a very successful French production. He saw it, and since the play is about music and Nazis, he offered me *The Pianist.*

You have taken on such challenging subjects, in the last twenty years. Is it partly the challenge that whets your appetite? (I'm tempted to ask, "Do you get the work in part because no one else accepts the dare?") What, heading into that script, was the most challenging aspect of writing The Pianist?

I never use the word *challenge* because it applies to all writing. It's jargon which I avoid. (Sorry, but when an actor, for example, says he accepted the role because it's a challenge, you can be sure that what he really means is he needed the money.) I don't know why I get offered these things. I long for a light comedy or something easy.

The difficulty with *The Pianist* was preserving the detached tone and point of view of [Wladyslaw] Szpilman, the author of the book. Not to have a voice-over or invent a companion to whom he could talk.

Polanski has a reputation in the United States (whether deserved or not—probably largely due to Chinatown*) of being tough on everyone, including writers. Can you extrapolate from your collaboration with him, and talk a little bit about the ideal way you like to work with a director?*

Polanski was the best of collaborators. He was never tough on me. We never argued but thrashed things out in an adult and professional manner. We spent five weeks together, in a house outside Paris, working every day from ten to six, laughing a lot and enjoying our work. That is the ideal way of working with a director.

When you are writing a picture of such scope, with specific geographical settings—and I'm thinking here of Love in the Time of Cholera *as much as* The Pianist*—how much description of the setting do you put into the script? And do you visit the actual locations as part of your preparation for the writing?*

I put in whatever I think is necessary for the production designer, but more importantly what I think gives atmosphere and color to the reader of the screenplay.

I seldom visit locations.

Dating back to A High Wind in Jamaica, *where Spanish is spoken by many of the characters (without subtitles!), your films cross language borders at will. You have worked with leading directors of several different nationalities. May I ask, how many languages do you speak or read? And how many languages you write in?*

One. English.

I gather you've set foot in Hollywood off and on over the years. And then you won the Oscar for The Pianist! *But of course most of the films that you do are the kind that would seem anathema to the Hollywood that reigns over American (and our exported American) culture. Do you have the feeling, when you go to Hollywood, of stepping into a den of iniquity? Or, over the years, have you developed a psychological (as well as real) distance from Hollywood?*

I get on well in Hollywood. The people in the industry whom I meet are serious and professional. But if anyone talks about "art" I run a mile. I like film gossip. I like keeping things light. I preserve the serious side of my nature for my work. Hope that doesn't sound too pompous.

Now, to Being Julia, *a film I loved. It was good to have an excuse to read the novella* Theatre, *one of Maugham's that I had not got around to. It must have been the lighter subject you were longing for. But not everyone would read that novel and say, "This could be a film!" Can you tell me a little about the genesis of your involvement in the production?*

Years ago I wanted to acquire the rights to the novella myself but discovered the Maugham estate was extremely complicated. I have very little patience and so let the thing drop. Then, a young producer, Mark Milln, who had never produced a film before and with very little money, acquired the rights and came to me. I said yes and wrote the screenplay. We had a tough time trying to get the film made until Robert Lantos, the Canadian producer, read the screenplay and decided to make the film.

Not everyone would think of Annette Bening to play the lead—a Midwesterner, American, et cetera. When you are writing a script, are you ever thinking of possible stars? Does it help, or hinder the writing at all?

I never think of stars and I never write for actors. To write for an actor is to imagine the actor's reality, not the character's, and that is, for me, disastrous.

As you have been a longtime close collaborator of the director of Being Julia, *were you involved in the casting at all?*

We had only done one film before, *Taking Sides.* No. I wasn't involved in the casting. But Annette Bening was an inspired idea. She is a superb actress and a star. Her age and looks were absolutely right, and to my mind was the best possible casting. I was disappointed that the distributors, Sony Classics, didn't do more to promote her chances for the Oscar after her nomination.

The book is really a marvelous character study. Without changing it greatly, finding things to use or emphasize, you shaped it so beautifully into more of a rounded story. I love how you brought the producer from the backstory of the novel into the script as someone who comments on Julia's "performances" throughout, much as Maughaum uses her parenthetical thoughts in the novel. But I also enjoyed the small touches not in the book ("T-O-M"); and things like her remark that there didn't seem to be any great parts for women anymore, because there were too many men writing the plays. I searched the novel, but couldn't find that line. It's yours, right? I know you mean it as ironic humor, but the same thing seems all too true of film, not enough female writers at the top of the field. Why is that?

Yes, those lines are mine. It's a constant complaint. I have no idea what the reason is.

I also enjoyed the writer-character at the end of the film, who is scarcely mentioned in the novel. He is misbehaving on opening night and getting drunk to overcome his nerves. Is that you at all? Are you nervous ever, still, about how your work will be received? Say, at a film premiere?

No, it's not me, but it is based on playwrights I know. I am less nervous now than I used to be. Age calms one. I seldom go to film premieres, as I have usually seen the film before the premiere and I know the end product will always be the same.

When I read the American reviews of Love in the Time of Cholera *I wondered if film critics understood "adaptation," or whether they actually read the book as most claimed. I remember one complaining that the tone of the film was "Dickensian." (Exactly right!—Latin Dickens.) The film hardly got a chance in U.S. theaters.*

I wonder if you might say something in general about your approach to adapting, drawing on the experience of Love in the Time of Cholera, *an impossible book to adapt for film, yet you did so marvelously. Are there certain steps you go through with any book? Are there certain things you are always looking for that will guide you and yet set you free?*

I think some of the reviewers simply wanted to make sure their readers knew that they had read the novel.

There are, for me, two important aspects to adapting. The first is what you are going to cut from the original work. The second is point of view. In *Cholera* I decided to cut the long opening sequence surrounding the suicide of Dr. Urbino's friend. The incident is never referred to again. That decision freed me to start with the parrot and the doctor's death.

I tried to tell the story from two overlapping points of view, that is, from both Florentino's and Fermina's points of view. But that was reduced to one—I think wrongly—because of the budget, I was told, but I think there may have been other reasons which I don't want to explore.

There were other sequences—one in particular, floating in a balloon across cholera-stricken country—that were also cut for budgetary reasons.

I would guess that was your most difficult adaptation, as there was so much to choose from and so many devoted readers lurking. Am I right?

No, I don't think it was the most difficult. *The Diving Bell and the Butterfly* was by far the most difficult. There is no plot, no obvious imperative in the progression of the story, and then, most daunting of all, there is the problem of the point of view. How could an audience be asked to gaze on a man in that awful physical condition for two hours or more?

I was stuck for about three weeks, almost telephoned the producer, Kathleen Kennedy, to tell her she had made a mistake offering it to me, when the idea popped into my head that the story should be told from Jean-Dominique Bauby's point of view. The moment I wrote the opening scene of him waking up in his hospital bed and typed the words: THE CAMERA IS JEAN-DOMINQUE BAUBY, KNOWN AS JEAN-DO, the screenplay more or less revealed itself. The story I decided to tell was the one of his illness, from waking to death, keeping the added little twist of how and when he suffered his massive stroke for near the end.

Though it is a deep book it is very slender. You had to invent a lot. You really captured his "voice." That might seem obvious as the book is in first person, but I mean you really captured a personality as well, which is not exactly the same personality in the book. Did you research the man himself at all? Or was it all drawn from your imagination and the book?

I did not research the man much. I met the mother of his children and his children who were guardians of his flame. I drew entirely from the book.

The female characters in particular I'd like to ask you about. I love that you made the amanuensis also the "butterfly," which is not the case in the book. The subplot of the mistress (not visiting him in hospital) versus the mother of his children (so diligent—and then that wrenching scene where she must answer the phone call for him, and it is the mistress). Were these people (the mistress and the mother) drawn from any reality you investigated? The women really enriched the film and also complicated the character of the man.

Everything was inspired by the book. The strange thing was that all the women—the physiotherapists, for example—were all beautiful. That is just a fact. I met one of them and was told about the beauty of the others by the mother of his children.

I invented the scene where the mother of his children interprets the mistress's call. I really do want to make clear to you that I seldom do a lot of research. I am not a journalist. I believe that the imagination is more reliable than research.

Once again, it is such a visual film; often the visuals are all we have except for the voice-over. I wonder if you can give me an anecdotal example of how something particularly visual, having to do with the main character's eye problems, evolved either from your reading of the book, or from discussions with the director—and how, then, you set it down on paper.

I took the scene where the eye is stitched up from the book and dramatized it. By making it from Jean-Do's [Jean-Dominique Bauby's] POV I hoped it would be for the audience painful and unbearable—which I am told it was.

[Director Julian] Schnabel must be given credit for the visual excellence of the film. But he and I had almost no contact. We do not get on. He is of the auteur school of filmmaking and not a very agreeable collaborator. In fact, I don't think he believes in film as a collaborative art form—which, of course, it most certainly is.

What can you tell me about how, and to what extent, you have gotten involved in this new Baz Luhrmann film Australia? *I notice the sometimes unreliable IMDb.com lists several writers, and it's my guess that you don't "collaborate" very often these days except with directors.*

Well, I did collaborate with Baz Luhrmann. He asked me to read a screenplay with which he wasn't entirely happy. I much admire his filmmaking and so decided to work on it with him. We worked in London, Paris and L.A. I had a highly enjoyable time.

I take your point about imagination as opposed to research or journalism. Why though, if imagination is the key, do you focus so much on adaptations in your work, as opposed to originals (with the exception of your own original plays and books, later adapted to film)? Is it partly the problem of convincing a producer of the inherent value of an original (as opposed to a presold title already known to the public)?

Adaptations need imagination, too. But if I have an original idea, my first instinct is to write it for the theater, which is my natural habitat. Furthermore, I haven't the patience to set up a movie.

I know this is a big question, but do you have any idea what, long ago, was so instrumental in nurturing your imagination? And do you have any habitual ways of coaxing it on a day when it feels like not working?

My imagination is always at work and I don't need to "coax" it. I like to sit in a restaurant, for example, imagining the lives of those around me. My wife joins in. Great fun.

My imagination was stimulated when very young, aged six or so. My mother sent me to what were then called elocution classes (she hated the South African accent and wanted us to speak decently). My teacher, Sybil Marks, gave mime classes—nothing stimulates the imagination more than mime. You have to imagine other objects, other people and make them real.

Many children's games require that sort of imagination. As I was the youngest of three children—my older brother was seven years my senior—I had what psychiatrists call only-child syndrome. I played a lot on my own. Also reading, the theater, and movies are wonderful stimuli. I have lived in the world of imagination all my life.

How do you choose from all the projects that are offered to you? What do you look for or think about foremost in terms of the job? Is there anything you wouldn't do? (I remember Julius J. Epstein answering this question firmly: "A Western, because I can't take them seriously.")

Yes, I wouldn't do science fiction because it is often very silly and sometimes too frightening. I was terrified by *Alien* (1979), and I had to run out of the room while my children went on viewing with no qualms whatsoever.

The subject on offer has to move me in some way—to laughter, to tears, to thought. I like to enter a world I have previously known little about or revisit a world to learn more. I think most important of all the characters have to have LIFE.

Do you write scripts with the same tools that you always wrote scripts? Whether yes or no, what are those tools? Longhand, typewriter, computer? Coffee, tea, or anything else at hand?

I started writing in longhand. Then the typewriter and, since 1982, the computer. Lots of coffee, and lots and lots of cigarettes.

What is the ideal time and place for you to be writing?

I can write anywhere—on top of a bus, if necessary—but I like to start at around 9 A.M. and work through until 1 P.M. I have a nap in the afternoon (read for thirty minutes, sleep for an hour), then go back to work but usually only to read and correct what I have written in the morning. But I never stop when stuck, always when I know what comes next.

February 2008

RONALD HARWOOD (1934–)

1962 *The Barber of Stamford Hill* (Caspar Wrede). Script.
Private Potter (Caspar Wrede). Script.

1965 *A High Wind in Jamaica* (Alexander Mackendrick). Co-script.

1966 *Drop Dead Darling / Arrivederci, Baby!* (Ken Hughes). Co-script.

1968 *La ragazza con la pistola* (Mario Monicelli). English adaptation.
Diamonds for Breakfast (Christopher Morahan). Script.

1970 *One Day in the Life of Ivan Denisovich* (Caspar Wrede). Script.
Eyewitness (John Hough). Script.
Cromwell (Ken Hughes). Script consultant.

1975 *Operation Daybreak* (Lewis Gilbert). Script.
1983 *The Dresser* (Peter Yates). Producer, script.
1985 *The Doctor and the Devils* (Freddie Francis). Script, based on Dylan Thomas's script.
1991 *Cin cin / A Fine Romance* (Gene Saks). Script.
1994 *The Browning Version* (Mike Figgis). Script.
1995 *Cry, the Beloved Country* (Darrell Roodt) Script.
2001 *Taking Sides* (István Szabó). Script, based on his play.
2002 *The Pianist* (Roman Polanski). Script.
2003 *The Statement / Crimes contre l'humanité* (Norman Jewison). Script.
2004 *Being Julia* (István Szabó). Script.
2005 *Oliver Twist* (Roman Polanski). Script.
2007 *Love in the Time of Cholera* (Mike Newell). Script.
The Diving Bell and the Butterfly (Julian Schnabel). Script.
2008 *Australia* (Baz Luhrmann). Co-script.

Television credits include "The Barber of Stamford Hill" (episode of 1960 series *ITV Television Playhouse*), *Evita Peron* (1981 telefilm); *Tales of the Unexpected* (twelve episodes, 1979–81 series); *Een familie / A Family* (1981 Dutch telefilm); *The Deliberate Death of a Polish Priest* (1986 telefilm); *Mandela* (1987 telefilm); *Breakthrough at Reykjavik* (1987 telefilm); *Countdown to War* (1989 telefilm); *Garderober* (1997 Yugoslavian telefilm); *Majstor* (2002 Yugoslavian telefilm).

Published work includes *George Washington September; Sir! The Guilt Merchants; The Girl in Melanie Klein; Articles of Faith; Sir Donald Wolfit; C. B. E.: His Life and Work in the Unfashionable Theatre; The Genoa Ferry; New Stories 3: An Arts Council Anthology* (as editor, with Francis King); *Cesar and Augusta; One Interior Day: Adventures in the Film Trade; A Night at the Theatre* (as editor); *The Ages of Gielgud: An Actor at Eighty* (as editor); *All the World's a Stage; Mandela; Dear Alec: Guinness at 75* (as editor) and *Home.*

Plays include *March Hares; Country Matters; The Good Companions* (libretto); *The Ordeal of Gilbert Pinfold; A Family; The Dresser; After the Lions; Tramway Road; Interpreters; J.J. Farr; Ivanov; Another Time; Reflected Glory; Poison Pen; Taking Sides; The Handyman; Quartet; Goodbye Kiss; Mahler's Conversion;* and *See You Next Tuesday.*

Academy Award honors include winning the Oscar for Best Adapted Script for *The Pianist*, and being nominated in the Best Adapted Script category for *The Dresser* and *The Diving Bell and the Butterfly*.

Winner of BAFTA in the Best Adapted Screenplay category for *The Diving Bell and the Butterfly* and nominated for *The Dresser*, *The Browning Version*, and *The Pianist*.

Writers Guild honors include a nomination for Best Adapted Script for *The Diving Bell and the Butterfly*.

NOTES

1 The well-known British novelist Martin Amis, then a young boy, plays a key child character, John, in *A High Wind in Jamaica*.

2 Wilhelm Furtwängler was a great classical conductor who compromised himself by staying in Hitler's Germany.

INTERVIEW BY **WILLIAM HAM**

JOHN HUGHES STRAIGHT OUTTA SHERMER

If you haven't heard of *Reach the Rock* (1998), you're not alone. In fact, considering its short, unheralded existence, you may well be alone if you have. Directed by newcomer William Ryan, it's a quiet, rather low-key (the less generous among us might call it "dull") character study of an overgrown delinquent (played by Alessandro Nivoli), stuck in a dead-end Illinois town, who spends most of the picture's hundred minutes breaking in and out of the town jail, breaking windows, and generally tormenting the slow-witted police sergeant who locked him up (William Sadler). Not exactly the stuff of blockbusters, and indeed, it died a quick and barely noticed death in 1998 as Universal, struggling with some of the worst business/timing decisions in its history (the words *Babe: Pig in the City* will chase several key execs to their graves, no doubt), dumped it in a total of three theaters in three cities for one week for a total gross of $4,960.

We could say that it's a worthy film that doesn't deserve to be forgotten, but nahh, let's be straight: it's because the dead-end Illinois town is a mythical burg known as Shermer, and, if you grew up young, confused, and full of nonsensical slang in the 1980s, you know the founding father of the town is one John Hughes, the man who best articulated the social stigmata of the misfit adolescent in the age of Chess King clothes and Keith Forsey–produced soundtrack records. After a series of phenomenally successful comedies that either (a) dealt with the mundane miseries of youth; (b) featured John Candy; or (c) both, the demographics that made Hughes the Tycoon of Teen, as synonymous with his time as Phil Spector, turned its back on the writer-director, and he contented himself in the 1990s with a run of slap-shtick farces featuring younger and younger protagonists (a trend that thankfully ceased after *Baby's Day Out:* God only knows where he would have gone from there ("*Wriggly Field!* The adventures of a misfit gang of Chicagoland spermatazoa!"), and remakes of old Disney films (an ironic turn for a man who ended his most famous short story by shooting Walt Disney in the leg).

Meanwhile, dozens of young filmmakers were pledging their troth to the Hughes oeuvre, and the next generation of Hughes boys were doing their best to keep Dad cool (the *Reach the Rock* soundtrack, on son John Hughes III's Hefty Records and featuring Tortoise's John McEntire and bands like Polvo and Poster Children, is by far the coolest collection of its stripe since *Pretty in Pink*—and no Nik Kershaw covers, either). John Hughes, still writing prolifically, became kind of reclusive. Thus one is humbled to be granted an audience with the man who defined modern teen cinema in all its flawed, erratic, awkward glory. (And if there happens to be any young adults out there named Duckie, Blaine, or Farmer Ted, you now know who to blame.)

. . .

Reach the Rock *is a very stark picture. Most of it takes place at night in a basically empty town, there's only about a half-dozen characters in it, very little action; it certainly runs counter to what sells tickets in this day and age. Why did you take that tack?*

I was just tired of the huge blockbuster-effects movies. I always liked character stories best—put two or more people in a room and get them talking; that's the whole reason I got into this in the first place. I'm not really a digital-effects–sci-fi kinda guy; I respect that when it's done well, but it's not really my cup of tea as a filmmaker, or a writer. If you look back at the films I've done, they take place over a maximum of three days and usually in a single setting. Even my road pictures are getting a couple of people in a car, then out of the car, into a room, and back in the car again.

It's interesting to me that you returned to Shermer after all these years, to find a much bleaker and less hopeful place than it was in the high school setting. Do you recognize the kind of character that Robin (Alessandro Nivoli) represents? Some part of yourself that never quite escaped, perhaps?

Not me so much as people I've known. It's a situation a lot of us can understand: you leave high school very quickly, time passes; ten years later you remember it a little more fondly than it might warrant, so you go back to a reunion or something and look at the people you knew for this short time in a particular place; you see how some have changed, and some might not have changed at all.

Now this guy [Robin] . . . you can go to any town and find these guys who never got around to leaving town; you can find them at the same bar they were at five, ten years before. It's a type I'm very familiar with from the community I moved to, on the North Shore of Chicago. There was a naval station in the town, so you had these "base kids" that would go to my school for a couple of years before they got transferred out. These were the real outcasts, fairly tough kids because of all they've had to put up with, completely outnumbered by the rich kids—it was a fairly affluent community, so you'd have these guys in the khaki pants and the Brooks Brothers shirts; if you were a cool guy, you could carry your books in one hand. Well, I always preferred to hang out with the outcasts, because they were cooler; they had better taste in music, for one thing; I guess they had more time to develop one with the lack of social interaction they had!

Then there were a lot of farm kids, who wound up in town because of community expansion and business muscling the farms out, so they went from being rural communities to being bedroom communities; and these people, the indigenous people if you will, wound up at the bottom of the social ladder because of it—lost in suburbia. John Bender [Judd Nelson in *The Breakfast Club*] was very much one of those characters. I think [Robin] is almost as if Bender had stayed with Claire [the Molly Ringwald character] at the end of *The Breakfast Club* and had never moved on.

It's the same with the locals in a lot of these resort towns: it's interesting to see how these small communities really get co-opted by money; people sweep in and say, "Let's bring all of our own kind of people, have our run of the town, and leave at the end of the summer." It really changes the face of these towns, and constantly so. I'm from Detroit, originally, a community that's been basically the same since 1920, and to come into an area that changes so constantly like that, with the original people growing fewer and fewer, is kind of shocking.

The whole notion of Shermer came out of that heterogeneous kind of society, very extreme—I mean, at one point, I went from a school with eleven hundred students to one with thirty. I remember this one kid, an eighth-grader, who had his teeth rotted out. *Eighth grade.* It was like *Deliverance* (1972). But then at the same time, you'd have the richest kid in town in your school as well, so even in this tiny setup, you had both ends of the economic spectrum, real extremes. I've always wanted to write a history of Shermer, because it'd be kind of the history of postwar America. Haven't got around to it yet, though.

And yet in a funny way, Shermer's a place that so many of us think of fondly. My teen years were defined to some degree by your movies, and I think a lot of people my age and younger can say the same.

Well, it was a great time in my life too, and I'm grateful, because it's that audience that kept me in business all those years. The studios never perceived those films as hits; they'd always bring them out in February, which is when the studios usually dump the movies they have no confidence in. Of course I was naive. I thought, "Fantastic! Right in the middle of that long stretch between Christmas and spring break; your coats are getting dirty, everything's dark, dingy—what a great time for a movie!" Especially one that's a little depressing. You see, one of the bits of wisdom I've picked up about adolescence is that joy and sorrow are equally pleasant to a teenager; those extreme states of mind are pretty cool whatever they are!

I think one of the reasons my movies have held up so well for as long as they have is that I've always tried to be true to my memories of the experience and show that on film. At the time I came along, Hollywood's idea of teen movies meant there had to be a lot of nudity, usually involving boys in pursuit of sex, and pretty gross overall. Either that, or a horror movie. And the last thing Hollywood wanted in their teen movies was teenagers! I mean, look at them—it was all twenty-five-year-olds in those movies. When I did *Sixteen Candles,* all the extras—the kids on the bus and in the gym—they were all real freshmen boys and girls from the same high school. [Anthony] Michael Hall was a freshman; the sixteen-year-olds were actual sixteen-year-olds, except for Molly [Ringwald], who was a year younger. You may not realize it now, but it had never really happened before, for very simple reasons: it's more expensive and harder to use kids. You only have four hours a day to shoot because of labor laws, but the results were worth it, I think.

Before you got into screenwriting, you were an editor at the National Lampoon *for several years; and before that you were like the Kevin Bacon character in* She's Having a Baby*—working in advertising, hoping to be one of the few to break out. That must have been quite a leap of faith.*

No, the real leap of faith was going for the advertising job! I had never finished school, so I'd go into these agencies and they'd ask, "So, where'd you go?" and I'd say, "UniversityofArizona" *[mumbling the words all run together]*. "Oh, really? What degree program did you do?" "Uhdidn'tgetthroughthere" *[ditto]*. "Well, thanks very much for coming in!"

But it looked really easy to do, advertising, so I put together this fake portfolio of stuff, they liked it, and I started freelancing once I broke in. Advertising was fairly simple work, and I really just wanted a job where I could sit and write every day and not get fired for it like I had at other jobs. But it was fun, I liked it, riding in on a train every day, all the travel . . . I used to go to New York every Wednesday for six years, because I had a client there. It got so I knew every flight attendant on the Chicago–New York route, and I started hanging out at the *Lampoon* offices on Madison Avenue. This was right at the tail end of the [editor] Doug Kenney era, *Animal House* (1978) was about to come out, P. J. O'Rourke was about to become editor-in-chief. I stuck around and, finally, I made someone laugh and they decided to keep me.

Getting into the *Lampoon* was like a Boy Scout initiation or something; they'd be very cruel to you until you made someone laugh, then they welcomed you into the fold. As it turned out, my timing was perfect, because once *Animal House* came out in the summer of 1978, breaking all sorts of box-office records and so on, Hollywood, in their infinite wisdom, came knocking and gave every writer at the magazine a development deal, including myself. I looked at that, thought, "Hell, this is easy," and flew out to Los Angeles and got four more development deals like that. Again, it's Hollywood jumping on the hot property; tell them you just got a deal, they'll want a part of you unseen. "We want to offer you a deal." "Hey, great, I just got two this morning!" I went back home, and there was a gigantic snowstorm in the winter of 1979, couldn't leave the house for two weeks; so I just hunkered down and wrote. It was great, and I haven't stopped since.

After the first couple of "adult" movies you wrote (National Lampoon's Vacation, Mr. Mom), *you seemed almost to stumble into the "teen angst" genre at exactly the time we needed it. I'm amazed at how quickly you became synonymous with the form.*

I had a very particular strategy for the timing of those movies, which I kind of had to educate the studios about. I told them, "I'm gonna grow an audience," which they didn't think I could do, but I did it. First of all, I tried to line up the release of each new movie with the video release of the previous one. That way, the first one might not do so well at the box office, but people would become familiar with it by the time the second came out, and so on. That's why my movies would come out every six months or so, and if you look, you'll see that the grosses steadily increased with each one. So I grew an audience, and I tried to be as true to that audience as possible, play to what they like and appreciate.

You know how, when you're a kid, you love it when you get mail? You feel important, like someone's paying attention to you. Well, we used to do that; every time someone wrote a fan letter to one of our cast members, every piece of mail that came in, we'd put their names on our mailing list and mail out huge packages every time a new movie was about to come out; kind of like what Disney does now—posters, rolls of stickers, all sorts of neat stuff. In fact, the only official soundtrack that *Ferris Bueller's Day Off* ever had was for the mailing list. A&M was very angry with me over that; they begged me to put one out, but I thought, "Who'd want all of these songs?" I mean, would kids want "Dankeschöen" [performed by Wayne Newton] and "Oh Yeah" [performed by Yello] on the same record? They probably already had "Twist and Shout," or their parents did, and to put all of those together with more contemporary stuff like the [English] Beat—I just didn't think anybody would like it. But I did put together a seven-inch of the two songs I owned the rights to: "Beat City" [performed by the Flowerpot Men] on one side and . . . I forget, one of the other English bands on the soundtrack . . . and sent that to the mailing list. By 1986, 1987, it was costing us thirty dollars apiece to mail out a hundred thousand packages. But it was a labor of love. I cared about my audience, and I cared about these movies.

You may have noticed I never sequeled them, nor did I want TV shows made from any of them. The only sequels I was involved in were under duress. I was only involved in the third *Vacation* movie, for example.

But you're credited as co-writing the second one.

Only because I created the characters. I didn't write any of it.

I must admit I'm relieved to hear you say that.

But the studio came to me and begged for another one, and I only agreed because I had a good story to base it on ("Christmas '59").[1] But those movies have become little more than Chevy Chase vehicles at this stage. I didn't even know about *Vegas Vacation* until I read about it in the trades! Ever since it came out, people have been coming up to me with disappointed looks on their faces, asking, "What were you thinking?" "I had nothing to do with it! I swear!"

Same with the TV shows. I tried to talk them out of doing *Ferris Bueller* as a series—talking to the camera is real hard, a lot harder than it looks, and I knew it'd never work, but they didn't listen. After that, they left me in the dark on these; *Uncle Buck* I knew nothing about until the producers asked me if they could use some of the exterior footage, establishing shots from the movie. That's when I got to put my foot down: "No fuckin' way! I'm a DGA member! Go get your own!" Then there was the time I was sitting at home, watching TV, and this commercial comes on for this new show. I'm watching it, thinking, "Jesus, they ripped me off. This looks just like *Weird Science*."[2] Imagine my surprise.

You haven't done a "teen" movie in a decade or more, but those really seem to be the films that are nearest to your heart, not to mention the audience's.

That was just a great moment in time for all of us. Apart from the real pleasure I had in just making up stuff, I thought it was great to have something for the young audience. I love writing young characters, and everybody can relate to a good teen movie; it's more immediate, honest, and there's a sense of group dynamics in that setting, that I prefer. A good cast of course helps—I'm not a big fan of "movie stars"—people whose handlers come up to you saying "We have to change the script . . . "—but then again, it's been about ten years since I've worked with actors who knew their lines! And by that I mean that they've studied the scripts for a while and internalized them to the point that they can play around a little, improvise on set and make their own imprint on the material. [Anthony] Michael Hall was very good at that, as was John Candy; they didn't care if they screwed things up a little because they'd usually screw them up in interesting ways. That said, I like young actors because they're so unspoiled, not like some of those actors who are about half an hour into their fifteen minutes of fame by the time they get to me.

I get the impression that you're not too fond of the Hollywood way of doing things.

I'm not, you're right. That's why I've stayed in Chicago, because I never quite fit into L.A. It's easier to maintain a degree of innocence here; you're not playing the herd so much. Even my biggest successes, like *Home Alone*, cut against the grain somewhat. Around the end of the 1980s, the studios wanted me to do something commercial—my old demographics had dwindled; there wasn't really an audience for the kind of stuff I used to do at that point. I'd never worked overseas with a really big star; Matthew Broderick was about as big as it got. They forced me to bow down a little bit. So I said, "Okay, I'll write a movie with a nine-year-old as the star, that'll show 'em" *[laughs]*. Little did I know . . .

I love some of the little details that get into your movies, that show up on screen for a couple of seconds and then are gone. One of my favorites is the shot of the Shermer sign in Weird Science *with the town motto—"One of America's Towns."*

I've always loved the movies where there are layers of different things going on at once, different things going on in the background while the main action's playing up front.

For example?

Well, was there a scene in *Planes, Trains, and Automobiles* in the bus station where . . . *[pauses]*.

Wait a second, don't you remember?

I don't remember if it made it into the released version! There are three-hour cuts of both *Planes* and *The Breakfast Club*, both of which have things I hope will surface one of these days. Anyway, in *Planes* there's a scene at the bus station: Steve Martin and John Candy are in the forefront of the scene, but behind them and to the side a little bit there's a guy with a shoebox in his lap, with all these white mice in it, coming in and going out quickly, just scurrying around for no good reason, except that I thought it'd be funny; maybe you're watching it for the third or fourth time on cable somewhere, your eye wanders away from the main activity in the scene, and . . . "Are those mice?" *[laughs]*. I must say I love that.

Before we wrap this up, I have a question about something that's been bugging me for fifteen years now . . .

"What's the punchline?"

To Bender's "naked blonde / salami / poodle" joke [in The Breakfast Club*]? No, I know better.*[3] *Same movie, though. At the end of* The Breakfast Club, *the criminal gets the prom queen, the jock gets the basket case, and the brain gets . . . to write the paper? What's up with that?*

Well, [Anthony] Michael Hall and I talked about this pretty extensively while we were making the movie. Other than the obvious technical matter, which is that there were five people in the film, so somebody had to get left alone at the end, we decided that Brian [Hall's character] was smart enough to know that wasn't on his agenda. He was the intellectual superior of the others, and it was enough for him to be accepted by them; that they'd think enough of him to let him represent the group on paper. I think Brian was intellectually mature enough to realize that he wasn't socially mature enough to handle a relationship anyway.[4]

That sounds like a massive rationalization to me, which my inner fifteen-year-old geek tells me would be just about right.

Sure! That's where that whole "girlfriend in Canada" thing comes from, which I used twice. "Oh, you wouldn't know her, she's in Canada." That way, you get to dodge the issue and still impress people—ooh, Canada, exotic. I like to keep that wavelength open, to stay in touch with the way kids think and feel, which is why I love talking about those movies. They're so near and dear to me. It's like being at the kids' table at Thanksgiving; you can put your elbows on it, you don't have to talk politics. No matter how old I get, there's always a part of me that's sitting there.

March 1999

JOHN HUGHES (1950–2009)

1982 *National Lampoon's Class Reunion* (Michael Miller). Script.

1983 *Mr. Mom* (Stan Dragoti). Script.
National Lampoon's Vacation (Harold Ramis). Script.
Nate and Hayes (Ferdinand Fairfax). Co-script.

1984 *Sixteen Candles* (John Hughes). Director, script.

1985 *The Breakfast Club* (John Hughes). Producer, director, script.
Weird Science (John Hughes). Director, script.
National Lampoon's European Vacation (Amy Heckerling). Story, co-script.

1986 *Ferris Bueller's Day Off* (John Hughes). Producer, director, script.
Pretty in Pink (Howard Deutch). Executive producer, script.

1987 *Planes, Trains, and Automobiles* (John Hughes). Producer, director, script.
Some Kind of Wonderful (Howard Deutch). Producer, script.

1988 *She's Having a Baby* (John Hughes). Producer, director, script.
The Great Outdoors (Howard Deutch). Producer, script.

1989 *Uncle Buck* (John Hughes). Producer, director, script.
National Lampoon's Christmas Vacation (Jeremiah S. Chechik). Producer, script.

1990 *Home Alone* (Chris Columbus). Producer, script.

1991 *Curly Sue* (John Hughes). Producer, director, script.
Career Opportunities (Bryan Gordon). Producer, script.
Dutch (Peter Faiman). Producer, script.
Only the Lonely (Chris Columbus). Producer.

1992 *Beethoven* (Brian Levant). Co-script (as Edmond Dantès).
Home Alone 2: Lost in New York (Chris Columbus). Producer, script.

1993 *Dennis the Menace* (Nick Castle). Producer, script.
Beethoven's 2nd (Rod Daniel). Characters (as Edmond Dantès).

1994 *Baby's Day Out* (Patrick Read Johnson). Producer, script.
Miracle on 34th Street (Les Mayfield). Producer, script.

1996 *101 Dalmations* (Stephen Herek). Producer, script.

1997 *Flubber* (Les Mayfield). Producer, script.
Home Alone 3 (Raja Gosnell). Producer, script.
Vegas Vacation (Stephen Kessler). Based on his characters (uncredited).

1998 *Reach the Rock* (William Ryan). Producer, script.

2001 *Just Visiting* (Jean-Marie Poiré). Co-script.
Beethoven's 4th (David M. Evans). Characters (as Edmond Dantès).
New Port South (Kyle Cooper). Executive producer.

2002 *Maid in Manhattan* (Wayne Wang). Story (as Edmond Dantès).

2003 *Beethoven's 5th* (Mark Griffiths). Characters (as Edmond Dantès).

2008 *Drillbit Taylor* (Steven Brill). Co-story (as Edmond Dantès).

Television includes *Ferris Bueller* (1990 television series based on his characters); *Uncle Buck* (1990 series based on his characters); *Weird Science* (1994 series based on his characters); *National Lampoon's American Adventure* (2000 telefilm, based on his characters); *Home Alone 4* (2002 telefilm based on his characters).

NOTES

1 "Christmas '59" was published in the December 1980 issue of *National Lampoon.*

2 *Ferris Bueller* did make it on the air as a (terrible) series on NBC, running for thirteen weeks from 1990 to 1991. (Perhaps the most interesting aspect of the show is that the part of Ferris's sister was played by an ingenue named Jennifer Aniston.) *Uncle Buck*

made it on the air around the same time (1990–91), with Kevin Meaney in the John Candy role. Seventeen episodes were filmed, eight were aired. *Weird Science* made it to television too, the USA Network. But you can't really call that one short-lived; it actually lasted five seasons (1994–98)!

3 Here's the joke, told by Judd Nelson's character (to himself) as he's crawling through the ceiling to get out of "solitary": "A naked blonde walks into a bar with a poodle under one arm and a two-foot salami under the other. She lays the poodle on the table. Bartender says, "I suppose you won't be needing a drink." The naked lady says . . ." He then falls through the ceiling before he gets to the punch line. Nelson apparently ad-libbed the joke on camera; there is no actual punchline.

4 Interviewer's note: Hall's character writes the paper the group was assigned at the beginning of the film, explaining just who they think they are, which, as someone who resembled that character more than any of the others at the time, always kinda cheesed me off—not only does he not get a girl like the others do, he gets all the work palmed off on him. Damn you, Hughes! Damn you!

INTERVIEW BY **PATRICK McGILLIGAN**

DAVID KOEPP SINCERITY

David Koepp was bemused at my suggestion that his small-town Wisconsin roots might help to explain the populist touch of a writer who has worked on as many Steven Spielberg films as anyone, and counting. As many Brian De Palma films too, for that matter.

But Koepp is not easily categorized. He is a writer who wears several hats jauntily. One of his specialties is "giant movies," which are usually adaptations of best sellers, classic comic books, or vintage television shows whose titles are already well known to the public. His "giant" scripts have launched several series and franchises with phenomenal box-office grosses and auxiliary revenue. At the same time Koepp stubbornly (he says "rigorously") alternates these remunerative blockbusters with his own "small movies"—sometimes adaptations, sometimes originals—chamberwork-type scripts that he writes "on spec" and, increasingly, prefers to direct. He also dabbles in short films (*Suspicious, All Falls Down*) that draw raves from IMDb.com reviewers.

To add to the mix of qualities, this quintessential Hollywood screenwriter chooses to live in New York City.

He started out as a theater major at Midwest colleges but finished at UCLA, where he relished the film studies program. After graduation he learned the ropes with independent productions (*Apartment Zero, Bad Influence*) before one of his scripts brought him to the attention of Spielberg. Hired before the age of thirty to co-write *Jurassic Park* (1993), he was launched into the top ranks of Hollywood writers and is still younger than most of his peers in the stratospheric salary bracket. Other megahits followed (*The Lost World: Jurassic Park, Spider-Man, Mission: Impossible*), while his "spec" side continued to evolve impressively. *Panic Room* (2002), with Jodie Foster and her daughter fighting for their lives from inside a secret room in a New York brownstone, was a nail-biter, while *Secret Window* (2004), which he adapted from Stephen King and directed, was a first-rate, intelligent suspense film, with Johnny Depp as an author stalked for plagiarism. His collaboration with Spielberg has now lasted over a decade. Most critics would agree that his script for *War of the Worlds* (2005), an expensive special-effects thriller with a compelling human dimension, was his finest yet for the director. At the time of this interview, he had just finished the third draft for another Spielberg project that was keenly anticipated by audiences.

. . .

I assume you grew up in love with movies, but at the time you grew up, and growing up in Wisconsin besides, there wasn't as much opportunity to see movies as there is nowadays—with avenues like Blockbuster and cable television.

No, there wasn't as much opportunity, so seeing a movie was kind of special. I remember one night when I was a kid—I don't remember how old I was, but pretty young—my mother said, "You can stay up late and watch this great movie on TV called *Notorious*." Just the idea that I got to stay up late to watch a movie was exciting and made it a special event. In those days when a great movie came on TV, you dropped whatever you were doing and plunked down and watched it, because you're right, you might not get another chance.

I also grew up Wisconsin, in Madison, and never saw movies growing up. It was unheard of. My parents wouldn't dream of spending the money and also, they thought movies were vaguely immoral. I really started going to movies and seeing too many of them in college at the University of Wisconsin. Was it the same for you?

That was when I started watching different kinds of movies, when I was in college in Madison. I saw a lot of film-society stuff and more foreign films that broadened my horizons a little bit.

We actually had a number of theaters around us, where I grew up in the small town of Pewaukee. There was the Lake Theater in downtown Pewaukee, which is now, I think, a discount store, but the marquee is still there. That was where I saw *Jaws* (1975) for the first time, even though my parents had specifically told me I was too young, but I was thirteen, and everybody else had seen it, and I had no intention of being a social outcast. There was the Park and the Pix theaters in Waukesha; I remember seeing *Annie Hall* (1977) at the Park when I was fourteen, and it blew my mind.

When I got in my later teen years, they built really nice theaters in Oconomowoc, The Scotsland Theatres, a few miles further down the road, where I have specific and wonderful memories of *The Shining* (1980) and *Star Wars* (1977) and *Return of the Living Dead* (1985). And as an older teenager, you could drive into Milwaukee, go to the Southtown Cinema, where I saw *Altered States* (1980) and a re-release of *The Exorcist* (1973), and I once broke up with a girl because she didn't like *Arthur* (1981). Of course a bit further into Milwaukee there was the Downer Theatre, which always had the best movies, bar none. I assume it's still up and running.

It's still one of the best theaters in Milwaukee, showing mainly independent and foreign films. So you managed to see a fair number of films, eventually.

I did.

Do you think coming from Wisconsin gives you a different perspective on writing scripts for movies, compared to all those Hollywood writers who come from New York or California?

It gives you *a* perspective, which is all you need. As a writer all you are is your bundle of experiences, and hopefully a point of view, which is one of the reasons why I think it's destructive for a writer to live in Los Angeles for too long, because then you're in the same cultural soup as everybody else and your ideas take on a certain sameness. Not to mention the corrosive value system there, where bad ideas are rewarded and good ones are punished. A system which I've benefited from and also suffered from.

You've got to come from somewhere, and then whatever your "you-ness" is, you bring it along with you wherever you go. In fact, it's all you've got.

Why did you go to UCLA? To get out of Wisconsin?

I spent my first year of college at the University of Minnesota. I was studying theater at the time, but it was a gigantic theater department, so I transferred to Madison, still wanting to become an actor. I spent two years in Madison, and I loved it. I really had a good time. I started working in a lot of plays and met people with similar interests, which is the great thing about college—when you realize you're not a freak. Or if you are a freak, that you're part of a subculture of freaks.

What was the height of your college acting career?

I think that I got to act at all was a small miracle, but the height of my illustrious career was probably when I played Mortimer in a main stage production of *Arsenic and Old Lace*. That was my triumph. I remember my review, actually, it said I was "brisk and efficient," which is better I suppose than "sluggish and sloppy." I've tried to remain brisk and efficient to this day.

But I was not very good at acting. I was plenty good for Pewaukee, but once I moved up to a slightly larger playing field, I realized there were a whole bunch of people who did it better than me, who, believe it or not, could go way beyond brisk and efficient. Also, I had started writing. I had always written since I was a kid, but around the time I was eighteen or nineteen years old I started writing movie-type stories in what I would later learn was the screenplay format. I soon realized that I wanted to write movies, and Madison did not offer a lot of filmmaking opportunities. I really needed a film school, and I needed to get out of Madison.

The only two real choices were New York or L.A., which meant NYU, USC, or UCLA. New York was tempting, because I'd always wanted to live in New York—as I do now, having finally moved here seven or eight years ago—but New York is not where the film business is. There's a filmmaking community here, of course, and plenty of movies get made here, but the opportunities are ninety-five percent in Hollywood, California, USA. So it didn't seem to make a lot of sense to start out in New York.

Between USC and UCLA, UCLA was public and USC was prohibitively expensive, so I concentrated on UCLA and then happily got in. One of the first classes I remember vividly was a film history class that met once a week for four hours, and you'd watch some great classic film in a perfect print, and then talk about it for two hours afterwards. The idea that this activity was in some way related to education, and that you could get credit for it, and your parents could say, "Yes, I see your going to school . . . " was just a mindblower.

Then there was film authors class, which met, I think, twice a week, and you'd watch, like, three Kubrick movies in one week—all great prints from the UCLA archives, on a big screen—and I'd never seen any of them before. Can you imagine, in one week, seeing *Paths of Glory* (1957), *Dr. Strangelove* (1964), and *Barry Lyndon* (1975), all on the big screen, all for the first time? It was incredible. Your jaw dropped. Polanski was another one we studied. I remember sitting through *The Tenant* (1976) and thinking it was the most amazing thing I had ever seen in my life and that I would get to do the same thing again tomorrow—see another Polanski film.

I would recommend film school just for *that* experience alone, the chance to take movies seriously and study and talk about them and meet a bunch of like-minded people.

Were you already concentrating on scriptwriting as an undergraduate at UCLA?

Yeah. You do a little bit of everything as an undergrad, and I did two years at UCLA—I was the five-year-program undergrad. But quickly you can decide where your emphasis is, and I decided it was screenwriting.

• • •

Initially, did you think you were going the independent film route, or was that partly accidental?

Initially I thought I would go whatever route would have me. I was really only looking for some way to pay the bills in the movie business, ideally involving writing them, but I felt it was presumptuous even to hope for that. Around this time I met Martin Donovan, an Argentine director who'd been living and working in Rome for years, and he was looking for an American writer to co-write a script with him. He'd read a script of mine called "Fatcity Upside Down," liked it, liked it a lot, and we really hit it off creatively. He had a lot of ideas, and we settled on what became *Apartment Zero.* Since we knew absolutely nothing about making a movie in Hollywood, we declared ourselves the producers, got help from a producer's rep, and managed to raise the money by hook, crook, credit card, and banked distribution deal. I learned more about making movies from that eighteen-month period than I have since. I ended up putting everything I earned for about two years into *Apartment Zero,* and though I never got anything back financially, I look at it as my very expensive postgraduate degree.

What brought you to the attention of Steven Spielberg? Because your credits are very good and solid before Jurassic Park, *but your early films really don't seem to be Spielberg-type films.*

It's a complicated story. At that point I had done *Apartment Zero,* which was a very quirky independent movie, and *Bad Influence,* also an independent, but really a studio thriller at heart. Martin and I had also written the script for *Death Becomes Her,* which was supposed to be an independent movie but ended up as something else entirely. Casey Silver, who was president of production at Universal at the time, had read *Bad Influence* and wanted to buy it, but he felt maybe it would be better as a buddy comedy. I thought that it wasn't actually a bad premise for a comedy, but said, "Since I've already written it as a thriller, can't we please make it as a thriller?" He said, "Um, I'd rather not, why don't you let us make it as a comedy?" I said, "Well, I think I'll go and try to make it somewhere else as a thriller . . . " So we ended up making *Bad Influence* somewhere else, and I think Casey liked that I had resisted an idea that I didn't think was right, so he called and said, "Why don't you come and write other stuff for us?" and I got an overall deal at Universal.

I dragged *Death Becomes Her* into the overall deal, and [Robert] Zemeckis read the script and wanted to make it, and then Spielberg was looking for a writer for *Jurassic Park,* so I think Casey recommended me. Spielberg read some of my stuff, we met, and I got the job.

Was that when you met Spielberg for the first time?

Yes.

Is personal rapport an important part of the equation with someone like Spielberg?

Sure. In meetings and in writing and in everything else you do in Hollywood, there's an incredibly important quality, which is sadly overlooked, and it's sincerity. You go to a movie and if they *meant* it, you can tell. You tend to like the movie. If they were pandering or trying to please you, or in any way insincere, you can feel it and you hate it. The same applies to meeting people. If you go to a meeting with someone and you have sincere feelings and enthusiasm about a project, or their work, or your desire to work for them, that's great. Not just hunger—sincerity. I always try to be in situations where I can be sincere, and if I don't have those sincere feelings, then I don't go, or hopefully I spot it in myself early on and don't pursue the situation.

One thing I have always admired about Steven is the sincerity of his enthusiasm has not diminished. It's safe to say Mr. Spielberg has had a fair amount of success, right? And yet in a meeting, he's sitting around talking about ideas with real sincere enthusiasm. The same with Brian De Palma. His enthusiasm is always heartfelt. He's one of the most cynical people on the planet, but not about a story idea that he likes.

Can you recall your first meeting with Spielberg? Here you were meeting someone whose movie, Jaws, *had thrilled and terrified you as a kid.*

Sure, of course, I was terribly anxious. That anxiety, though, diminished quickly—over a period of about twelve years *[laughs]*. It wasn't really until *War of the Worlds* that I stopped feeling uptight, and, I think, the result is the *War of the Worlds* script is probably the best one I wrote for him.

There's an anecdote Jean-Claude Carrière, Buñuel's scriptwriter, tells about being hired to work with Buñuel as a young man just starting out in film in the early 1960s. They'd have these long lunches together, talking over the scripts, sometimes with the producer sitting in . . .

I read somewhere he estimated he had two thousand meals with Buñuel.

After their second or third film together, the producer pulled Carrière aside and said, "You know, I hired you to say no to him once in a while."

[Laughs.]

Is it hard to say no to Spielberg, because of the anxiousness you mention and because of the awe and admiration with which any writer must first approach him?

It was at first, and it's easier now. But what I discovered after a while is I could say no—you can say no all you want—and don't worry about it. If he really wants to do something, he's going to do it.

After all, he's a writer too.

He's very much a writer. A storyteller. The situation is much like that of having a point of view—coming from somewhere, being someone, having some point of view. It's the same thing with your opinions. You're hired for your opinions. So they really shouldn't get mad at you when you express your opinion. But they do—that's part of the risk—and that's okay. You're still hired for your opinion.

It's like what the Michael Lerner character says in *Barton Fink* (1991): He says, "The contents of your head are the property of this film studio."

So Spielberg likes a give and take?

Sure. I think there's a calmness about successful people, because they know they can prevail. So he's fine with give and take. I don't think anyone likes to be *argued* with, but he does like give and take, and he enjoys it with the calmness of someone who knows that he's in charge. Ultimately the decision is his.

I remember in the second *Jurassic Park* film (*The Lost World*, 1997), there was one particular scene I was opposed to, and I'd argued against it like nine times but lost every time. But I just could never bring myself to write it, so I'd turn in draft after draft, and Steven would always ask, 'Where's the blah-blah scene?' And finally we were shooting, and the blah-blah scene was just a couple days away, and he was still asking for it, and I summoned all my nerve and told him I just absolutely did not want to write the blah-blah scene. And he was very sympathetic, and put a hand on my shoulder, and said of course, he understood, and he certainly was not going to force me to write it. "But when we *shoot* it, here's what I'm going to do . . . " And look, the thing is, that's how it should be. The director has to make his movie, he's a hack if he doesn't, and that's just the way it is.

Is there any way you can encapsulate what you bring to him that he can't get from some other writer?

No. I can't, really. That is a question better left for someone else. It's hard for me to say.

Obviously, you do, though.

It's been three movies and we're working on a fourth, so *something's* working.

Can you talk a little about the progress in script quality that you mentioned, from Jurassic Park *to* War of the Worlds*? Is it partly the differing nature of the material, and your own maturation as a writer, as well as the growing ease of collaboration?*

Hard to say, they both have their virtues and their inherent problems. I just think I did a better job with the characters in *War of the Worlds,* perhaps because there were fewer of them, or maybe because I was depicting a domestic situation that I thought I knew something about. Whether it's dinosaurs or alien invasions or some other gizmo, it is very, very difficult to get real human beings into these giant movies—sometimes the gizmo eats you, and sometimes you eat the gizmo. I just felt like on *War of the Worlds* I got to take a decent bite out of the gizmo.

Can you compare Spielberg with De Palma, in terms of your interaction with them, or your process of collaborating with them?

They're completely different human beings with completely different worldviews.

They are completely different. Normally, I'd think the same writer couldn't necessarily write regularly for both of them.

True. But aside from the fact that they view the world in hugely different terms, the actual process of collaborating is no different, I would say. With anybody you get along with and have a creative rapport with, the process is not really any different. You talk, you throw out ideas, you argue over them, you embrace them. It's all pretty much the same.

Do they both leave you alone to the same extent?

To varying degrees, and in different areas. They both have a huge amount of input into the story, of course, particularly in the more visual setpiece-type scenes. They both tend to keep their hands off the dialogue. They'll contribute, question, criticize, edit—but they'll never sit down and write lines, which I appreciate.

If you're a screenwriter, particularly for a visionary director or a director with a distinct and powerful point of view, you have to go in with the attitude that you're an assistant storyteller. It's the nature of the medium. You're there to help.

One similarity between the two is that, one way or another, you have specialized for them on scripts that are suspense, action thrillers, or stories with a springboard of tension, right? That's become one of your strengths and part of your reputation.

It's certainly the thing I like to write the most, but tension exists in every single genre. It's just that it's the most overt in suspense-type stuff, or adventure.

It's life or death in the films you've written.

But suspense can be tiny. One of my favorite suspense sequences in any movie is in *Quick Change* (1990), Howard Franklin's movie with Bill Murray. There's a scene where Bill Murray has to get away from some mobsters who are chasing him and who haven't yet realized he's there at the same intersection as they are. He runs to get on a bus, but Philip Bosco, who plays the bus driver, says, "You don't have the exact change. I can't take you without the exact change and this bus is leaving in sixty seconds." So Bill Murray runs into a Bodega to get change, but there's a very slow-moving lady in front of him in line, and meanwhile the mobsters start running out of the building across the street. The suspense is murderous, and it's all over whether the lady in front of him can pack her groceries quick enough for him to get change so he can get on the rules-fanatic bus driver's bus. The scene is hysterical.

. . .

*You have worked on so many franchise hits, series, sequels, and blockbusters—*Jurassic Park, Mission: Impossible, Spider-Man *and now* Indiana Jones*—is it really challenging, to put it nicely, to write on a project where there are so many hands trying to stir the pot?*

It's a whole different challenge, but yes, it is a challenge. The thing about a Spielberg blockbuster is you're usually only dealing with him, so that makes it easier, and that's why those are enjoyable. *War of the Worlds* was a great deal of fun for me, one of the most enjoyable writing experiences I've ever had.

Something like *Spider-Man,* there's a lot more people involved and therefore a lot more opinions and more possibilities for conflict. So that can be harder. Again, that's part of your job, but that's why I try to mix it up by writing originals, at least half the time. The résumé doesn't necessarily reflect that, as the originals are less likely to be produced—I've had six or seven of them made, and probably twice as many adaptations actually make it onto film. But whether they get made or not, I've tried to be rigorous about writing original scripts half the time.

If you want some peace and quiet, you've got to write on spec sometimes. It'll get noisy later. But that's really the only way to get peace and quiet. While if you take a job, you have to understand . . . you've taken a job.

Did you choose Spider-Man*—that is, were you a fan of the comic books, growing up—or did it somehow choose you?*

It was a job I was up for, and very, very much wanted. I had loved Spiderman when I was a kid, and it was clearly great material for a movie. The studio was clear with everybody that nobody just gets this job handed to them, you have to come in and impress us, it was an audition. So I did as much prep work as I could, and I found all the relevant sections of the various comics that I was interested in, and put it all up on big posterboards, and went in there and pitched my little ass off. Happily, I got the job. Never underestimate the power of office products.

Do you ever work with the important writing collaborators whose names appear on the franchise hits alongside yours, people like Robert Towne for Mission: Impossible? *Or is it always one after the other?*

It's always separate. It's always sequential. I guess maybe there are some people who are really big of spirit, who might be able to completely put their ego aside and collaborate with whoever they bring in, but I can't imagine that situation happening. Again, you're hired for your opinion. These are *your* opinions. If someone comes along and tells you to change your opinion, you can either do what they say, or you can go away. It's up to you. But to stick around and do something you don't believe in is really bad for the human spirit.

When you go to Guild social functions and run into someone like Robert Towne—this is hypothetical, of course—is there anything to be said between you about Mission: Impossible? *Other than to greet each other and chuckle?*

Not a lot. That one had a particularly snarky back-and-forth process that hurt my stomach lining. He's a fine human being, it's just that we were put in a position where we kept rewriting each other and that's not a great basis upon which to begin any relationship.

A snarky back-and-forth? So sometimes you write a draft, someone else takes over, but then the producers come back to you later on?

That happens quite a bit. You experience a little bit of the beaten-wife syndrome. You work for a while and you think everything is going good, then they fire you and you're angry, and they go away, telling you, "We're very sorry, but you made us do it." Then there's someone else for a while and it doesn't work out and they come back to you and say, "We're so sorry, please take us back," and you say, "Okay, just don't hit me anymore, please?" So you take them back and then they fire you again and you say, "You hit me again!" and they say, "But you *made* us hit you again!"

Do the stars have much input? Do individual stars ask for you? Because you've been writing a lot of heroic male leads—Tom Cruise more than once, for example. And stars like Cruise have a reputation for getting involved with the script.

I think any actor who is allowed to have a voice is going to want to have a voice. The good ones speak up about some things and step back and let you do your job about the other things. I think the writer is almost always the choice of the director or the studio, sometimes they'll run it by the star, but he or she rarely initiates that choice, unless the film is further along and there's some sort of distress.

But I don't usually do those kind of "distress" rewrites. I haven't often been in the position of reading somebody else's script and making changes that the stars want. I usually start from scratch. I like to start fresh and stay on a project through to the end. Those two-week production polishes I've done once or twice, but not often.

Is that one of the virtues of working with someone like Spielberg, that even top stars are deferential to him?

It's nice to have someone in charge. Pretty much all the guys that I've worked for—Spielberg, De Palma, David Fincher, Bob Zemeckis, Ron Howard—all the really good ones have been squarely in charge. That's good for a movie because, again, it gets back to the question of point of view. It has to be somebody's.

I love Panic Room, *incidentally, and especially on your list of credits it stands out among a lot of films with male leads as a film with a really strong female lead. Otherwise, you seem to be specializing in heroic men.*

That's true. I'd like to write another great female lead. I wrote that one on spec.

You did?

Yes. I read an article in the *Times* years ago about "safe rooms," they're called, and I ripped it out and threw it in the story-ideas file, and I didn't think about it again for a couple of years, until I moved into the townhouse in New York where I currently live. The building had an elevator, because the person who lived here before was disabled and had this elevator installed. It's an old, creaky, slow elevator, and I was riding in it one day, just thinking—looking through the cage gate, watching the floors move by as the elevator went up—and I started thinking it would really be fun to do a contained-space thriller that was vertical instead of horizontal. Then I remembered that old article and started to write.

My initial idea was to write a "bottle," a real contained-space thriller with rigorous rules, such as: "We can never leave the house" and "Absolutely minimal dialogue."[1] I think when you restrict yourself in certain ways, you end up creating interesting boxes to write your way out of. I also wanted to try a new approach to outlining, so I wrote a thirty-page treatment first, and then the script. After so much prep, the first draft of the script only took a couple weeks.

Fincher was the first and only director ever in on it, and we were initially making it with Nicole Kidman, but after a couple weeks of shooting she blew her knee and had to drop out. So we were lucky enough to get Jodie Foster to step in.

It's great that you write scripts on spec. The franchise films give you that freedom, but a lot of people don't jump at the opportunity.

Because there's a downside. I wrote a spec last year that hasn't sold, for example. So you can spend four or five months on something and have it come to naught. I think we will make that movie some day, but it's been tricky. If you say to yourself, "Well, I could take this job and absolutely get paid," or, "I could write a spec and maybe get paid and maybe get nothing," human nature being what it is, you're going to lean towards the job.

I'd think you wouldn't need the money at this point. That you could afford the four or five months it takes to write a spec.

It's not just about money. With a paid job, you're on something you know the studio is interested in because they called you up. Sometimes there are interesting people involved, like an interesting director, or an interesting star, or a powerful producer who is going to be an ally. So there are a lot of reasons.

Can't you take a short cut and pitch the spec idea?

Pitches suck. Pitches are a drag. Other than *Spider-Man,* I've never had a pitch that worked out well, because somehow they heard it differently than what you said. Or you said it in a way that implied something it's not. Any time you pitch something and they say, "Oh yeah, we'll buy that!" by the time you turn it in either the person who bought it has been fired, or the person who bought it says, "Oh, *that's* what you meant?" By then it's too late because you've already accepted money and there you are—stuck with a person that didn't want your movie in the first place, or at a studio that wanted something else entirely.

As long as you're going to go to the trouble of putting together a good pitch and flying out to California and meeting with a bunch of people and hawking your wares, the amount of time and trouble that takes, it doesn't take that much more to write a first draft. Then you can be absolutely clear what it is, and besides, a script always ends up somewhere you didn't imagine. Whoever you thought would love it can't stand it, and somebody you never dreamed would be interested thinks it's great. If all goes well. Of course, sometimes they all hate it.

This spec script you just wrote—can we talk about it generally, without giving away the idea or story. When you started it, did you foresee the obstacles they put up, once it was completed? Or does the process of writing and selling a spec script have an unpredictable life of its own—and, each time, all the problems reinvent themselves?

Every script has its own problems and you never know what they are, going in, and you are continually humbled before the process of storytelling. You can't learn enough about it, and you can never really get too good at it. You can develop a lot of skills. You can develop ways to finesse your way out of problems, but good, clean, simple storytelling is like writing a catchy pop song. It's a completely mysterious process—occasionally they drop from the clouds, but usually they don't.

So you're not blaming the problems with selling a spec script on the nature of the industry and the fact there are only a certain number of production slots.

Well, sure, there's that too, and if you handed me an excuse like that I'd be a fool not to grab it. There is an awful lot of luck involved. *Panic Room* happened to come along at a time when they were interested in doing female-driven thrillers, so I benefited from that. I can't say I designed it that way, I just happened to get lucky. You can also miss that wave. I wouldn't want to be the guy that has a new superhero movie right now.

But you never know. You luck into stuff, or you don't. If you try to predict, you'll be chasing the parade rather than leading it.

• • •

How much do your problems with spec scripts have to do with your determination to direct your own films? It seems as though you are intentionally building a sideline of more chamberwork-type films that you want to write and direct.

That has a lot to do with it, because spec is the only way you control the material, unless you option a book yourself. Although the last two movies I directed both made money and did well and everyone made a profit, I'm clearly not the first guy you'd go to when you're looking for a director. But I'm *my* first guy, so if I control the material that helps.

In the 1930s and 1940s the writers who directed were few and far between—I think that was true all the way up into the 1970s. Do you think it should be de rigeur nowadays, or that it is good self-defense, for any young writer to aspire to direct? Or does it make perfect sense for a writer to say, "No, I'm not interested in directing."

There's a couple of reasons why it's not so common, still, for writers to direct. First, the jobs require completely different personalities. Writers and directors are just different human beings. You can have both sides of that in your personality, or not. I know several writers who I think should direct and I think would be good directors, but they have no interest in it because of the lifestyle, the heartache and sorrow and bullshit, and I understand that.

The lifestyle?

You have people in your face constantly. Most writers I know enjoy their time alone in a room. They don't necessarily enjoy the time writing, but they like the alone time *[laughs]*.

On the last movie I directed I finally figured out why directors wear baseball caps. It's so you can use the brim to avoid eye contact with people, because someone is always trying to catch your eye to ask you, "Should this be red or green?" and you just can't take it. You're usually busy trying to think your way out of some problem. There's a barrage of questions and beseechers, and it's hard to find a corner to crawl into.

Writing *and* directing, doing both jobs at once, is very lonely. You lose a vital collaborator. The good directors who are not threatened by their writers, they like someone who has the same creative stake in the process as they do. Someone who cares as much and has as informed an opinion. Plenty of people come along who don't have fully informed opinions, but you can't necessarily listen to them because they're not looking at the whole picture, or they haven't thought about it long enough. When you're a director and you have a writer you trust, it's a great relationship.

. . .

My guess is that someone like you wakes up every morning with a pile of books or ideas that have been overnighted to you by big important people and major studios who want to hire you.

I wish it were that way. I do get a fair share of offers, and I'm grateful for that. I worry about the day when it stops. But it's not quite the deluge you describe.

What makes you say yes to a book or idea?

I've always felt it's binary. It's either one or zero. You read something or you hear an idea, and either your head swims with possibilities, or it stands inert. If you have a lot of ideas and enthusiasm and, again, sincerity, then you should do it. If you don't, you shouldn't, because you're not going to work it up later.

What do you think of all the general negative criticism of Hollywood?

It's deserved. But we do get an excessive amount of scrutiny, considering our rather unimportant pursuits. Just trying to tell a few good stories, nobody's trying to hurt anybody.

But you said you too have suffered from the system. Is that why you moved to New York? Before I first got in contact with you I thought of you as the prototypical Hollywood screenwriter, but here you are in New York writing spec scripts.

There are plenty of prototypical Hollywood screenwriters living here—William Goldman, Tony Gilroy, Richard LaGravenese, Brian Koppelman . . . ; there's a lot of us here. I live here because I've always wanted to. When I was seventeen years old, I visited my brother for a couple of weeks after he had moved to New York, and I said to myself then, "I'm living *here!*" My search for a career took me to Los Angeles, and I stayed there a while—fifteen years—and then I realized I didn't have to live there, I could live where I wanted to live. So I came to New York.

What I was trying to say earlier is that Hollywood tends to reward not so original ideas and withhold reward from good ideas. That system I've benefited from greatly. I think I've had some not-so-good ideas and not-so-good scripts that were lavished with praise and reward. But I also know I've had some good ideas and good scripts that went unloved. That's the way it is. The trick to playing Hollywood is getting your good stuff through.

Which is why you can never really know a screenwriter, because you never know what they have in their drawer. A movie can come out that is questionably one of the worst movies ever written. It's not just that they screwed up the writer's script; maybe the script was never that good to begin with. But the guy who wrote it might have a masterpiece in his drawer that no one will let him make.

What is the difference in style and format between the scripts you were writing as an amateur—before you ever sold one—and the ones you are writing nowadays?

In style and format they haven't changed a lot. I formed a style I liked when I was about twenty-two. I started reading scripts at that age, and it impressed me, first and foremost, that this had to be a reading experience, because these are awkward documents that are half of something. They are meant to simulate another experience, which really doesn't happen anywhere else in art. A song is a song. A novel is a novel. A painting is a painting. They can all be taken at face value. A screenplay is meant to simulate another form of art, and that's tricky.

So I realized that things have to be read at a certain pace, because movies don't slow down and speed up; they keep moving past you. The action may slow down or speed up, but the rate at which it goes past you is always the same. So you've got to replicate that pace on the page, and keep the reader moving without stopping. I came to a style that I thought helped that problem, and that hasn't changed a lot. It may be a little more exaggerated now than it was then, because as you grow older you become who you are—only more so. But it hasn't changed a lot.

Can you characterize your style any further? Wordy, epigrammatic?

I can be wordy, although I try to save it for bursts, or wordiness when absolutely necessary. I do like white space, though, because I don't think there's anything more depressing than turning a page and seeing densely formed paragraphs. I also found that I end up usually doing one sentence as a shot. Or a paragraph is a shot. And I use a lot of dashes. I'll begin a sentence with one line, like, "He opens the door"—then, dash, dash—new paragraph—dash, dash—"There's a huge monster." You know what I mean? Because that implies the rhythm of what's going to happen. A guy opens a door; you can picture it, and you know something suspenseful is about to happen because there's *dashes*—why else would the writer put these ridiculous dashes all over his page? Maybe *There's a huge monster* is underlined, or in *italics*, or some poor invention to simulate something special happening on screen.

What's your next script that will be produced?

You *nev-er fuck-ing* know *[laughs]*. There are a couple of originals I'm trying to direct, and I adapted a remake of *The Taking of Pelham One, Two, Three* (1974), for Sony, which I think they're going to do. The original was a brilliant script by Peter Stone. It certainly had to change, though, because the world has changed in the last thirty-three years, particularly New York. But I tried to be very respectful of his script.

Will there ever really be an "Indiana Jones 4"?

I sure hope so. I sure hope so. I feel like the script's gone very well but there are a lot of powerful opinionated people involved, so who knows?

Is there any tiny morsel of information you can tell me about the story or script?

The main guy has a bullwhip.

September 2006

DAVID KOEPP (1963–)

1988 *Apartment Zero* (Martin Donovan). Co-producer, co-script.
1990 *Bad Influence* (Curtis Hanson). Script.
1991 *Toy Soldiers* (Daniel Petrie, Jr.). Co-script.
1992 *Death Becomes Her* (Robert Zemeckis). Co-script.
1993 *Jurassic Park* (Steven Spielberg). Co-script.
Carlito's Way (Brian De Palma). Script.
1994 *Suspicious* (David Koepp). Director, script (short film).
The Paper (Ron Howard). Co-producer, co-script (with his brother Stephen Koepp).
The Shadow (Russell Mulcahy). Script.
1996 *Mission: Impossible* (Brian De Palma). Co-story, co-script.
The Trigger Effect (David Koepp). Director, script.
1997 *The Lost World: Jurassic Park* (Steven Spielberg). Script.
1998 *Snake Eyes* (Brian De Palma). Co-story, script.
1999 *Stir of Echoes* (David Koepp). Director, script.
2002 *Panic Room* (David Fincher). Producer, script.
Spider-Man (Sam Raimi). Script.
2004 *All Falls Down* (David Koepp). Director only (short film).
Secret Window (David Koepp). Director, script.
2005 *War of the Worlds* (Steven Spielberg). Co-script.
Zathura: A Space Adventure (Jon Favreau). Co-script.

2008 *Indiana Jones 4* (Steven Spielberg). Script.
Ghost Town (David Koepp). Director, co-script.

2009 *The Taking of Pelham One, Two, Three* (Tony Scott). Uncredited contribution.
Angels and Demons (Ron Howard). Co-script.

Television includes *Hack* (creator and executive producer of the 2002 series); *Suspense* (director and executive producer of 2003 telefilm).

NOTE

1 *Bottle* is storytelling slang for a story confined in terms of time or space, as in "a ship in a bottle."

INTERVIEW BY **TOM MATTHEWS**

RICHARD LAGRAVENESE A WRITER UNDER THE INFLUENCE

Born and raised in Brooklyn to parents who shared with him their love for movies, Richard LaGravenese was hardwired to appreciate the intricacies of filmmaking from a very early age. He spent much of his youth absorbing the classics, in front of the family television and at the theater. "When Gene Hackman is about to run into the woman with the baby carriage in the chase scene in *The French Connection* (1971), it happens right across the street from the Loew's Oriental, which was a huge, art-deco movie palace. That's where I saw many of the movies that I loved."

Spending his nights with the likes of Bette Davis, Olivia de Havilland, and Ingrid Bergman, LaGravenese matured into a writer with a particular knack for capturing the voices and inner lives of women. He specializes in high-profile book adaptations and the under-the-radar polishing of scripts on the verge of production (his uncredited work on *Erin Brockovich* is known within the industry to have been critical to the film's success). With *Living Out Loud* (1998) he made the leap to writer-director, recently directing Hillary Swank in the romantic comedy *P.S. I Love You* (2007). In 2003, he and the late Ted Demme produced and directed the acclaimed documentary *A Decade under the Influence,* a bracing tribute to the films and filmmakers who defined American cinema in the 1970s.

A firmly entrenched New Yorker, LaGravenese sold his first script, *The Fisher King* (1991), as the industry came out of the 1988 screenwriters' strike, and he was interviewed for this collection on the eve of the 2007 work stoppage. In between, he rose to the top of the A-list, working among that rarefied group of writers who are offered virtually every hot project in town and who have the luxury of choosing only those assignments that stir their passion. LaGravenese enjoys professional status and financial rewards far beyond what was afforded the writers who crafted the classics that showed him the way.

. . .

Given that you were born in 1959 and came of age cinematically amid the critical triumphs of the early '70s and the blockbuster era shepherded in by Spielberg and Lucas, I'm surprised you didn't approach screenwriting until your late twenties. That was actually late in life given the youth movement of the times.

At the earliest age, before I was a teenager, movies were my lifeline. I didn't play sports very well and Brooklyn was kind of a hostile atmosphere, and movies were really the escape and the safe haven for me. As I got older, theater became something that I began to explore and really love. Eventually my career goals were more toward theater, thinking that movies were something so far away that they weren't something that I would be able to get close to. Whereas being from Brooklyn, New York and theater were right there. It was something that I could touch and feel and be a part of.

What was your taste in movies when you were a kid?

I loved old movies. My parents had me at a late age, so their movies were the movies of the '30s and '40s. My mom would let me stay up until one o'clock in the morning because some great Bette Davis movie was on, or some classic. When I was a little kid and she would describe a movie to me, especially those movies from the '30s and '40s, I would think, "My god, I *have* to see that." I don't know if it was because of the way she described them, but the best of those movies ended up being movies like *Dodsworth* (1936), *Notorious* (1946), *All about Eve* (1950); those are the movies I remember her telling me that I *had* to see.

Your father also encouraged your passion for film.

My father was a real sports fanatic and I was his only son, but I wasn't into sports. We didn't have a connection there, but he would take me to the movies every Sunday. It being the late '60s and early '70s, the rating system was just then changing and he never cared about whether they were rated R or whatever. He would take me to see things like *The French Connection* (1971), *The Godfather* (1972), and *Marriage of a Young Stockbroker* (1971). He took me to see *The Wild Bunch* (1969) when I was nine or ten because William Holden was in it; he didn't realize that it was going to be a Peckinpah movie *[laughs]*.

So I had this balance between classic movies and what were then contemporary movies. Back then, there was "The Million Dollar Movie" on local New York television, but there was also the four-thirty [P.M.] movie.

And then because my father worked the late shift as a cab driver, sometimes we'd watch the late show.

Did your father always choose the movies you saw in the theater?

He usually chose the movies we saw together. But I was a huge Jerry Lewis fan when I was a kid, so on my own I would always see his movies. I could go to the movies alone when I was nine or ten years old. I was a latchkey kid, and back then it was okay to do that.

I was into comedies. I loved Neil Simon. I remember seeing *The Odd Couple* (1968) at Radio City Music Hall. I would see anything I could get my hands on, it didn't matter what genre they were. For some reason, I remember as a kid I saw *Husbands* (1970) three times, and I don't know why. But I was fascinated by that movie.

Did you and your father talk about the movies?

I remember him talking to me very excitedly during *The Godfather*, because in Brooklyn *The Godfather* was a major deal. I remember him in the balcony of the Loew's explaining to me what was going to happen. Everyone who was Italian-American in Brooklyn felt like they knew the inside scoop on that movie.

He took me to see *Where's Poppa?* (1970), which I remember being hysterical, but he was so angered by it because of the language. I remember loving that movie.

You were shaped by the movies of the '30s and '40s, and of the late '60s and early '70s. Are there common traits to those eras you can identify?

The acting. The really great performances. I was always intrigued by great acting. I was conscious of the great directors of those older films. William Wyler was one of my favorites as a storyteller and for his ability to get great performances out of his actors. He always intrigued me when I was young.

I also loved the "kitchen sink dramas" of the '50s. I loved Elia Kazan, Delbert Mann, Robert Wise. There was a nice, dark '50s period I responded to.

Because of my background in theater, I also have a special affinity for plays which were made into films during those periods. Wyler did a lot of those, like *The Heiress* (1949) and *The Letter* (1940). Later films I loved were *Who's Afraid of Virginia Woolf?* (1966) and *The Lion In Winter* (1968), based on plays that were very literate. The writing in those are what really excited me.

Even as a kid you were conscious of the writing involved?

It was always the writing that got me, in all the genres. Everyone talked about *Notorious,* which everyone loves for Hitchcock, but Ben Hecht wrote that script. No one ever talked about the writers of Hitchcock's movies, but Hecht wrote *Notorious,* Ernest Lehmann wrote *North by Northwest* (1959), Evan Hunter did *The Birds* (1963)—these were great writers. So I think even without knowing it, it was the writing which was attracting me. I could always recall scenes. I was able to remember dialogue *exactly* the way it was done. After I saw a movie, I could recite the dialogue.

I remember seeing *Klute* (1971) and being so affected by the atmosphere of it, but I mostly remember lines from it. I remember that scene when the Jane Fonda character was trying to get the tape from her psychiatrist. When I finally met Jane she told me that a lot of that stuff was improvised, but the way that it was done in such a nonwriting style impressed me so much.

When you revisit those old films, do they hold up? Did the eras in which they were made enhance their appeal?

Sure, but if you look at *Dodsworth* now—which was made in 1937, written by Sidney Howard from a book by Sinclair Lewis—the writing is so good that the issues which it was dealing with then could be transplanted to today. It's the story of a woman who is afraid of aging and who wants to have flings, even as her husband is getting comfortable in their old age together. The way that Wyler shot a married couple arguing over these issues, there's a timelessness about it. But it was also ahead of its time.

The kind of work that Bette Davis was doing holds up today. She could be very arch in some of her performances, but she did less than a lot of the stars of that period were doing. She did a better job of reflecting how people really behaved, even though she could sometimes be very flamboyant or too mannered at times.

How about the films of the '60s and '70s? Do any show their age?

What amazed me when I did *A Decade under the Influence* was the pacing of those films. When I had to pull clips for the documentary, which was my favorite part of the project, I would go to my favorite scenes and I couldn't believe how long they were. I had to reduce a lot of them because there was so much breath in them. The pacing was a whole different thing. And the subject matter, and the language.

Even *Save the Tiger* (1973), a movie which isn't as well known and wasn't a big hit, is an extraordinary script. Oh my god, I remember seeing it at the movies. And to make that movie now with a major star would be nearly impossible.

Waldo Salt, my god. I see *Midnight Cowboy* (1969) now and I am always surprised by how funny it is. It is one of the most depressing movies ever made, but it's also really funny. It is such a great script.

The films that defined you were also rich in dialogue, which is one of the things which you are now acclaimed for in your career.

Writing dialogue is my favorite thing to do, and it's the thing I remember most from those movies. Watching a [Joseph L.] Mankiewicz film or watching a Billy Wilder film, what I remember are scenes and dialogue. Not so much the visuals. As I've gotten older and started directing I am affected more by visuals, which is really interesting. I'm watching films now and thinking, "That's a really cool image, that's a cool visual." I used to never see that sort of stuff before.

When you're writing, how do you know when a dialogue scene is working? Do you speak the lines out loud?

Sometimes. There's a music to dialogue. I remember when I was nine years old I had a free period in school, and every day of that school year I would go up to the library and read *The Odd Couple* over and over and over. I just couldn't get over the music and rhythm of Simon's writing. The pacing of the jokes, the setup and the payoff.

So I think I learned through osmosis. I started to feel the timing. I still overwrite. I think a lot of my buddies who are writers overwrite. But the skill is in what to take away and how to find that perfect rhythm.

At what point do you begin to realize that what worked in your head is not necessarily going to work coming out of an actor's mouth?

Writing a screenplay is such an evolutionary process. When the actors come on board, and hopefully you've cast the best people for it, you hear the dialogue spoken out loud and you think, "Oh god, this is so overwritten. I don't need half of this."

I remember on *Bridges of Madison County* there were some lines from the book that Clint [Eastwood] wanted me to use, and I remember being worried because I thought they were unactable. I had been an actor, and I know that if an actor can't deliver a line without it sounding weird, it's going to be clunky. But Clint is the most confident guy and had so much experience, and he said, "You know, it happens all the time. You read something on the page and it reads beautifully and it just doesn't work when acted; and then you read something else on the page and it feels like it's going to be clunky and it plays beautifully. We'll figure it out when we're on set." And that's what he did.

The Fisher King, *which earned you an Oscar nomination, was the very first script you wrote on your own. I understand that it evolved through a series of drafts which would be unrecognizable compared to the film that was ultimately made.*

The character of Jack [played by Jeff Bridges] was originally a burnt-out cab driver, a cynical guy who at one point had a lot of aspirations and hopes but was beaten down by the system. He meets this homeless guy, and in the course of their friendship he realizes that the homeless guy is an idiot savant, and he winds up manipulating him for his own purposes. I finished this draft, and then I picked up the *New York Times* and there was an announcement of preproduction on this movie called *Rain Man* (1988). It was exactly the same plot as my script, and I couldn't believe it. I didn't read scripts, I lived in New York and wasn't tied into the movie community, how the fuck did this idea get into the ether? Did I pick it up from someone else?

So I threw the whole thing out and started over: same two guys, but a completely opposite tone. The first version was very heavy and intense and pretentious, sort of what a first draft would look like from someone trying to be "important." The second draft was like a sitcom. I just went the whole other way and wrote something funny. Jack was an heir to a fortune and he was a layabout, and he hooks up with this homeless person. That draft didn't work at all; it was just a silly, nonsense draft that I didn't like, but out of it came the character of Lydia [played by Amanda Plummer in the film]. Jack had to marry off his girl cousin to get his hands on the fortune, and he decided to fix her up with this homeless guy. So now I had Lydia, and I started all over again.

What finally brought you around to the myth of the Fisher King?

I got turned on to a psychologist named Robert Johnson, who had written three books called *He*, *She*, and *We*. They were all about Jungian archetypal psychology, where he would take a myth and put it together with male psychology, female psychology, or couples psychology. And to help explain men, he used the Fisher King.

What was important for my story was that when the Fisher King was young, he was sent into the forest on a kind of vision quest. There was a sequence where he cooks a fish, and when he touches it it burns him. The way that Johnson interpreted this was that part of male growth is that at an early age, we have an experience as we're approaching adulthood. We sense our own power and connectiveness to something bigger: call it spirit, call it soul, whatever you like. But because we're young, it's an experience which overwhelms us and it burns us. It's a wound that we carry, and according to Johnson we spend the rest of our lives searching for that connection again. But in our culture, because we don't have rituals and spirituality, men tend to try and find that connection through making money, or having lots of women, or driving fast cars, or acquiring power.

Robin Williams's character calls himself Parry, although that is not the character's given name. That's your link to Parsifal of the myth.

Parsifal is an archetype of the Fool in a hero's journey, which is the part of us who will take the journey without questioning it. If you're cynical, if you're tainted by too much experience, you tend to not take chances, you tend to not go on adventures and journeys because you know too much. You sit back and you think about things and you analyze, and you decide that it's not going to happen.

Johnson wrote that every man has to tap into his Fool, that young, naive part of yourself that says, "I'm going to jump off that cliff even though I don't know what's going to happen, " or "I'm going to set off on this journey to find the grail, even if I don't know if it actually exists." You have to have that part of yourself to create. And Johnson was saying that you had to have that part of yourself to be a whole man. Only a fool would take the journey, and only the journey can take you to wisdom. So to be a wise man, you have to start off as a fool.

This is all fascinating, high-toned stuff, which I'm not sure was the smartest thing to pursue while trying to break into Hollywood in the late '80s.

Yes, but I was a fool, so I took the journey *[laughs]*! I had no idea what Hollywood wanted. I didn't read screenplays, I didn't go to film school. And I was being influenced by different sorts of storytelling.

Early on, before Jack's downfall, he's plotting his next career move and you have him nakedly express his desire to make the public know his face along with his radio voice. And then when the media seizes on the shooting that Jack provoked, it is his face which is all over the TV. A great "be careful what you wish for" character turn.

The weird thing is that when you click with an idea, those sorts of things just happen. I had never intended that moment you're referring to. But when an idea clicks, I believe that you begin to be guided, if you're open to it and you don't block it off by being egomaniacal or too controlling. You have to surrender to not always knowing where you're going, and allowing inspiration to guide you a little bit. It's uncomfortable, it can be really frustrating. But if you have faith and persistence and commitment to the idea, and the idea is *right*, you start to find some wonderful things.

There's a quote from Einstein which says that a problem cannot be solved with the same mind that created it. You've got to come at things with a completely different mind when you get blocked like that, and you have to be willing to throw out anything.

All these years later, it's still hard to believe that you hadn't developed the material with Terry Gilliam from the beginning, it so perfectly meshes with his sensibilities.

Terry had just had that terrible experience with Columbia and *The Adventures of Baron Munchausen* (1988). He hadn't had an agent up to that point in his career, he had always just developed his own work, but he had allowed CAA to come into his life to turn things around. His agent sent him two scripts. One was *The Addams Family* (1991), and the other was *The Fisher King*. He read my script, and he said that it felt like he had written it. It expressed so many ideas that he and I shared.

Gilliam is known so much for his visual style and sense of spectacle, while your script was very emotional and character-based. Was there any fear that the heart of the piece might be lost in his hands?

No, that was the beauty of it. What he brought to my world and what I brought to his world was a great marriage. Terry *is* a visualist; his art is his visuals, but when he directs he is all about the writing. He doesn't understand the sort of director who takes a script and dismisses the writer and goes off and does his own thing with it. He believes that if you say yes to a script that becomes the bible. You interpret it and do work on it, but *with* the writer. His joke, though, was that if the film didn't work, he could always say, "Don't blame me! *He* wrote it."

Do you recall any healthy differences of creative opinion with him?

Listen, I was just in awe of the whole thing. My personality doesn't include the healthy arrogance that many of the people I admire have. But he never took advantage of me in any way and we agreed on too many things for there to be a problem. We both agreed that we didn't want to make the movie that a lot of people would've wanted, which was the Capra version of the movie. He wanted to keep it as edgy as possible, although I hate that word. He didn't want it to be maudlin and sentimental.

Tell me about the genesis of the Grand Central Station sequence, in which commuters famously begin to waltz.

Early on, Terry kept saying that he was trying to get away from making this a "Gilliam film," and we were like, "No! We want you to do your thing, this is why you're you." So we were scouting the location at Grand Central, and I had originally written a scene where there was a homeless woman singing and people were giving her money. At this point in the story, Jack had lost everything, but he sees all these people in the terminal listening to this woman sing, and he feels a sort of bond with them. He feels part of this community, and senses the beginning of him coming back to life.

So we're up on the promenade looking down on the main floor, and Terry says, "Wouldn't it be funny if everyone just started dancing at the same time?" Everyone goes, "Oh my god, that would be amazing," and Terry says, "I was just kidding!" But it was so much better than what I had come up with. For Jack to start feeling a part of the community at that part of the story was too early. So instead of making the scene about Jack he made it about Parry's love for Lydia as he watches her move through the terminal. With that one visual idea you got to step into Parry's world and the romance of his vision.

But of course if the film had failed, that scene probably would've been another nail in Gilliam's coffin. Just one more mad, budget-straining visual idea which fell short.

But that's what makes him Terry Gilliam. And God bless him for it.

With the success of The Fisher King *you were hired to take on subsequent projects. How did* A Little Princess *come about?*

It was one of those projects that Disney had on the shelf and Mark Johnson was attached to it as a producer. At the time, he and Barry Levinson were very powerful producers, they had done *Rain Man* and *Tin Men* (1987), which I loved. I thought Mark would be a great person to work with and I had a young daughter, so I was personally in that place where the story appealed to me. I read the book, I read the script that Disney had previously done, I watched the old Shirley Temple movie [*A Little Princess*, 1939], and I decided I could bring something to the material. What I loved about the story is that it's about the power of imagination, about how this girl survives her experience through the power of her imagination.

You have since gone on to earn acclaim with a number of adaptations of novels. What did adapting A Little Princess *teach you?*

I think you have to have a point of view for the book. You have to decide what it's about, and that becomes your screenplay spine. From that, you can eliminate what you don't need to tell the story and you take what you do need. And because it's going from one medium to another, sometimes you invent new material.

What did you learn in the early days about working in Hollywood?

The first project I did at Disney was one of those classic experiences where I was in development hell for draft after draft after draft. These were in the years when there was Michael Eisner and Jeffrey Katzenberg, and you'd get sixteen pages of executive notes that just went on and on and on. The first project that I said yes to was called *Widows*, which was based on a British TV series written by Lynda LaPlante. I think I was in development on that for over a year, and that was the first time I thought, "This *can't* be the way this works."

When I did *Little Princess*, it was getting to that point again and I finally stopped. I learned how to say no after too many notes. They said that no director wanted to do the script as it was, but I stood my ground and said that if they found a director *then* I'd make more changes. It ended up just laying there until Mark Johnson took it to Warner Brothers and it got made there.

A film that you did get made at Disney was The Ref, *starring Dennis Leary, Kevin Spacey, and Judy Davis, and directed by Ted Demme. Apart from it being such a dark film for the studio, it was surprising to see Don Simpson and Jerry Bruckheimer's names as producers. They were known for big-budget, high-concept summer movies.*

The Ref was based on an idea by Marie Weiss, who is my sister-in-law. I brought the idea to Disney and guaranteed it, which meant that she would get to write it, and if work was required I would come in and rewrite.

I would also be producing it with my brother-in-law, Jeff Weiss, but the studio wanted one of their in-house producers involved as well. We ended up hiring Simpson and Bruckheimer because we figured they were the least likely to be like the "corporate" kind of Disney producers. I think they were interested in the project because of Dennis Leary, who at the time had a big MTV presence. Which caused a mistake in the marketing because they tried to sell it to teenagers when it was really more for adults.

There came a point where Judy Davis was growing unhappy with her character in the development of the script, I think due to some of Don Simpson's notes. She was really upset at the first table read, but I said, "Don't worry, I work fast, I can get this back on track." I would sit down with Teddy, the actors, and Jerry Bruckheimer to go over the script, and then I'd go home and write forty pages for the next day. And that continued throughout production.

It was pretty great to make such a dark film for Disney, although *The Ref* still has a heart. That's part of Dennis's gift, in that he can make highly unlikable characters funny and sympathetic. That's where his humor comes from.

The film did not do well, which one always worries gives studios ammunition next time someone pitches them a dark film with "unlikable" characters.

Well, they released it in March instead of at Christmas, and they marketed it to teenagers instead of the adults who would've gotten it, so there were a lot of reasons why it didn't do well.

Another project which evolved from the early heat your earned from The Fisher King *was* The Mirror Has Two Faces, *which was ultimately directed by Barbra Streisand in 1996. I recall hearing that it began in the early '90s as something else entirely.*

It was based on a French film [*Le miroir à deux faces,* a 1958 film directed by André Cayatte], which TriStar had bought as a comedy for John Candy. TriStar had just made *Fisher King,* which hadn't come out yet, so I watched the French version and came to them with a different take, a romantic-comedy take.

Le miroir à deux faces *was not a comedy. The heroine is transformed through plastic surgery, leading to the murder of her doctor by her husband. What inspired you to take it in such a different direction?*

When I was in the fourth grade, I wrote this short story. I think it was the first original thing that I ever wrote. It was called "James Bond and the Girl with the Buck Teeth," and it was all about James Bond being paired with a female partner on a mission. She's unattractive, but he falls in love with her anyway. And I feel like I've been writing the same story ever since. I have this fascination with what beauty is and how in a relationship someone can start out being not that attractive to you and then because of who they are, you fall in love with them and they *become* beautiful. Or conversely, as you get to know people who are extremely attractive they can become ugly. It's all in the eye of the beholder. So this was something I wanted to explore in *Mirror*.

Honestly, I feel that *Mirror* was something which I never cracked. I wrote four different versions of it, and I liked the third version the best, but it was the fourth version which got made. I did a version where she doesn't get plastic surgery, and I did another where she does. In one version the surgery changed her personality, in another it didn't. In the third draft, I came up with a character who represented that lover who comes in and out of your life, and you're so in love with them that every time they leave they break your heart, and when they reappear they can open you up again. You have no immunity to them. And that's why in that draft the Jeff Bridges character decides that he wants to have a loveless marriage, because he's so obsessed with this woman that he can't put himself at emotional risk. But I just never felt like I cracked that version.

Was Streisand involved when you first took the job?

No, nowhere near. She became involved around late '91 or early '92. We met because *The Prince of Tides* (1991) and *Fisher King* were both up for a lot of the same awards, so our paths crossed. She had a lot of reservations about doing *Mirror*. She was very aware that the material was something she had already explored in the early part of her career. She was very unsure about whether she wanted to just direct it and not appear in it, or if she wanted to do it all. But she and I had a similar interest in exploring how love works. How much of it is attraction, and how much is something else?

There's a backstory to this which I want to express. In Brooklyn, where I come from, Barbra Streisand was one of the biggest icons in the industry. For everyone in my family, she represented that person from Brooklyn who made it across the river to New York. And she did it in such a big way. She was so unique and such a huge talent, but she didn't look like everybody else. She made it out of pure talent and guts.

I remember when *Funny Girl* (1968) came out. Back then you had to go into the city to see big releases; they wouldn't come to Brooklyn for several months. So when *Funny Girl* came out, my whole family got dressed up and it was like an event. I was too young at the time, so my father took me to see it alone after that. And I remember thinking how unique it was that this actress and this character had kind of fused, where you couldn't tell one from the other. Even before that, people forget the impact she had on television and in the recording industry. She was a huge talent.

When I went to meet her for the first time I had to call every relative in Staten Island and Long Island, and they were all flipping out. But I had this conflict. This was very early in my career, and the writer part of me was really pissed off at the fan part of me. I was this burgeoning writer who was trying to form his own ideas, but the fan part of me just wanted to please her and was intimidated by her. I had all this fan ideology to work through, and during our first period of working together in the spring of '92 it was very difficult. The project actually fell apart.

But then over the next couple of years, we both went through big changes. She started performing concerts again, which she hadn't done since the late '60s, while I did *Little Princess, Unstrung Heroes* (1995), and *Bridges of Madison County*. We came back together, and it was a completely different relationship. I remember her saying to me that I seemed so much more confident. I said, "Yeah, I am. I feel like we can relate on a more equal basis." And we had a wonderful time together.

There is the long classroom scene in the film, in which Streisand speaks at length about courtly love while the [Jeff] Bridges character observes her and is won over. Are those your words? Are they her words? How did that speech evolve?

We worked on that together. We did a lot of reading on the subject, and then had long discussions across the big desk in her house. For us it was addressing a core idea in the movie, and we spent a lot of time on it. But we definitely wrote it together.

Like some of the other directors I've worked with, she has a mind which is so curious about how things work. She loves to try to figure out how humans tick. I know that she gets a bad rap from some people, but I would defend her to anybody. I think she's great.

When the film came out and didn't do well, I felt terrible because I felt like I had let her down in the writing somewhere. I felt that she got unnecessarily attacked. I didn't think they needed to be as vindictive as they were.

A lot of reviews knocked Mirror *as a "vanity production," as if she initiated the whole thing to celebrate herself.*

Right, and she didn't initiate it. She was dragged into it kicking and screaming. That's what made me so angry. It was a subject she was interested in exploring, but it took years to get her to commit because she was reluctant to be a part of it. But the problems with the film were in the script, and I wish I had solved them.

The Jeff Bridges character is such an odd presence in the film. He reminded me of Henry Fonda in The Lady Eve *(1941), reducing romance to this loveless abstraction, but he doesn't quite work as a character. Once Streisand committed to play the female half of the relationship, is it possible that the male half of the equation didn't get as much attention in the development?*

It wasn't a question of getting equal attention. I just think as a writer who was still developing his skills I didn't nail that character, I didn't figure him out totally. I never came up with something strong enough to make you understand him. And, again, I take responsibility for that. I just didn't write him well.

Going forward, were you more aware of recognizing that moment or that character which you haven't articulated perfectly yet, and knowing when to put on the brakes until you have?

Just in the past year, I've learned that I have a lot of false beliefs about things, and one of those things is time. I have a false belief about how much time I have to work with, and how much time it should take to get things done well. There's a part of me who is that kid who just wants to get his paper turned in on time, but I have had to put that part of me in the corner and say, "No more." Everything gestates at its own speed. Now I am a little more brutal with myself. If something in my writing is not clear, then I should put the pen down until it *becomes* clear instead of just pumping out work and moving forward. If the problem is thematic, then I need to stop and consider things. And wait.

The Bridges of Madison County *was a huge publishing success and had been purchased for Steven Spielberg to turn into a movie. What was the status of the project when you went in to pursue the writing assignment?*

There was no director at the time. There had been two scripts done by two different writers. I read the book, and this was a case where I had to go in and say, "This is how I would do it." I told them that I would always tell the story from the [Meryl] Streep character's point of view and that I'd try to bring more of an arc to the story, which wasn't in the book. And I distinctly remember saying that the characters need to have a fight. I was raised by Italian women and I know that an Italian woman doesn't have great sex for four days and then just say, "I know you have to leave. Goodbye" *[laughs]*. She'd feel some kind of conflict. So that lead to the scene in the kitchen, which wasn't in the book.

Had you read the book prior to going after the job? Were you aware of the derision it was receiving in loftier literary circles?

Everyone had their opinions about that book, but it was a huge best seller. It was reaching women in a meaningful way, and I felt that there was something in it that could be told honestly in a movie. I asked my sister why she loved the book, and she told me that women get to a point in their marriage when they've been together for so many years and the kids are grown up and they begin to believe that they're never going to feel real passion again. You can be snobbish about the writing in the book, but the idea was something that was universal and it was touching women throughout the world.

In my first draft I went way off the book as I was setting up the Streep character. I wrote in her fantasies and things like that, but Clint was very smart. He said when you're working with a book that popular, you want to add to it and improve it, but you don't want to sacrifice what made it a success to the people who did like it in order to attract those who didn't. The trick was striking that balance between the two.

I had to write the story fresh, as if the viewer knew nothing of this story or these characters, while knowing that fans of the book knew all this already. People who knew the book knew that they don't end up together, but we created that moment at the end where you wonder if she is going to join him in his car and go off with him. I remember hearing that women in the theater were thinking for just that moment that she *is* going to end up with him, which I thought was great. We wanted the people who knew the book so well to have that experience of *maybe* getting a different ending and then giving them what they actually wanted, which was the ending in the book. If we had changed it too much, then people wouldn't respond to it. But we wanted to be able to surprise them. We wanted them to get so caught up in how we were telling the story that they believed that we might've taken the ending to a new place.

I remember before I started writing the script I watched *Brief Encounter* (1945). *Bridges* was like a foreign film in that way. It was very simple. It was a two-character study of a love affair. That kind of story is much more common in French or British cinema, so this was an American version of that. And Clint directed in a way which took its time.

Eastwood was not the first director on the project. He was preceded by Bruce Beresford.

Beresford fired me. I got the movie greenlit. Clint said yes to just acting in the film off my draft, so then they needed a director. That was at first Bruce Beresford, who threw away my draft and brought in Alfred Uhry.[1] They set up shop in Iowa and I didn't hear anything for two months, and then come June Beresford is gone and Clint is directing and he's bringing my draft back. The first time I met him was on the plane to Iowa to look at the set. A lot of the work was just reducing some of the stuff that I had added that was not in the book.

This was your first trial by fire on a high-profile studio project, the sort of assignment you have become known for. Did working under such pressure come easy for you?

I respond well to the challenge of coming onto these big projects and solving the big problems. It's going to sound really simple, but when you go in and you show excitement and enthusiasm and passion and a point of view, that goes a long way. When people come in—even a director who's auditioning for a job—and everyone's acting *cool,* it doesn't work as well. People really respond well to excitement and enthusiasm. That's why the projects you choose should be the ones you are enthusiastic and excited about, otherwise you have to fake it and that's torture. I tend to not take jobs unless I have ideas that I feel strongly about. I get offered a lot of things that I say no to because I don't have a feeling for them, even though they are big opportunities.

Your big break came with The Fisher King, *which was based on your original idea. After that, you primarily adapted novels or rewrote existing scripts. Did the assignment work take you away from developing your own material?*

At that point I was in my early thirties and I had never really had a real job. Prior to *Fisher King* I was doing survival jobs, I had never made more than $125 a week. I come from a lower-working-class family where money was tight, often through very tough periods, and now I had a family to support. So when I was being offered studio work, as opposed to taking a year off to write an original without knowing if it would ever get sold, I was happy to have the jobs. The key is finding a creative connection to the material where you can get excited and make it something personal for yourself.

That early experience was like going to school. I was working with great directors and I was learning my craft, and I was getting paid for it.

The Horse Whisperer *was quite similar to* Bridges*: a commercially successful if not critically admired "women's" novel, directed by and starring an iconic actor-turned-director. Eric Roth had already done work on the project; how did you find your role on it?*

I was offered the gig and I read the book. Afterward, [Robert] Redford and I had a conversation and I asked him, "Why do you want to tell this story?" It wasn't a sarcastic or insulting question but a genuine thing I needed to know: what was it about the material which made him so strongly committed?

He said that while he was raised in Southern California, he had lived and raised his family in New York and in Utah. Two places he loved, but two entirely different energies. One being urban, intellectual, stimulating, creative, and one being more connected to nature and of the earth. He saw the book as exploring those two dynamics, the western mind meeting the eastern mind. In describing the eastern mind, he said that when men live in places that they build, in concrete, they are less connected to the earth. They get a sense of themselves as being in control of life, as opposed to being a part of the rhythm of life. That sense of false control leads us to become neurotic because we really can't control life the way we think we can. That's what he thinks causes the eastern, urban mind to be more of a neurotic mind, which he saw in the Kristin Scott Thomas character in the film.

Then there was the western mind. I knew from my own experience with working with Native Americans that their whole rhythm is completely different. They work in conjunction with and cooperation with nature. They work with the earth and its cycles. Their sense of time is completely different from someone in the city, who thinks he can control time. The Native Americans wait as long as they need to wait until whatever they need to have happen happens. The character that Redford played was of that mind. He lived in closer connection to the wild, to nature. It gave him this healing sense which could heal that eastern mind. Bringing them together is what fascinated him. I thought that was a fascinating idea.

The interesting thing was that Redford and I *were* those characters. I was the eastern neurotic guy, and he was the western guy. I remember going to locations with him in Montana to the farm where they were going to shoot the movie. We drive in and there are all these cows staring at us, and I was afraid to get out of the car. They were cows, they were probably more scared of us than we were of them, but they were really big cows *[laughs]*.

Redford jumps over a wooden fence and I follow, and I get a splinter. He goes to this house that he's going to rent and there's a dog there, so Redford says hello to the dog. Then I say hello to the dog, and it jumps on me, rips a giant hole in my jeans. I told him that Montana knew that I was from Brooklyn and it was fucking with me. It was really kind of funny that my energy in that town was so out of sync, and that's who the Kristin Scott Thomas character was. I think that's what I brought to it.

I loved working with Redford. He's so smart about the script and he's so fun to work with.

He has a reputation for deliberating a lot as a director, sometimes to the frustration of the screenwriter.

I learned that when you're in collaboration with him, he's working things out as a director. He'll keep talking things out even though you think you've been over it already, but I realized that he's trying to clarify it in his own head. When I started directing, I realized that that's a great way to work. Especially when you have a screenwriter to work with.

A far different adaptation challenge was Beloved, *which was based on one of the most acclaimed novels of the latter part of the century and was being developed by Oprah Winfrey. The film was not the critical or commercial success that had been expected, which must have been disappointing.*

I had done the adaptation for Oprah and received this beautiful leather-bound copy of the book with an inscription from Toni Morrison, thanking me for the adaptation. I was very proud of it. It was the first time that I didn't impose any ideas onto an adaptation which didn't come from the book. *Beloved*, the novel, was such a beautiful piece of work that all I did was find a way to translate it to cinema, but the screenplay was all Toni Morrison. But I had a different way of looking at the material than the filmmakers, and there were sections of it that got lost. And when *Beloved* got greenlit at the same time as *Living Out Loud*, which was going to be my first film as director, I couldn't continue into production on it. They moved on without me, which often happens.

I thought the film lost some of the poetry from the book. I thought it was at times almost too literal. There were scenes and moments from Toni Morrison which I loved and which I had put in the screenplay that were cut and never filmed. I felt that they would've given the film more texture and human complexity. But who knows, I could be wrong. It's easy to judge after the fact. And when you're a screenwriter in love with a script, you can lose perspective.

The best movies are the ones where everybody is making the same movie. Jonathan Demme, who is one of my favorite filmmakers, had his vision of it. We had different ideas about it, and the fact that I had to leave anyway was probably fortuitous because he was able to continue with a different writer, my friend Adam Brooks, to convey his vision. You'd have to ask Jonathan how successful it was for him, apart from the box office or anything like that.

The official credits on a movie are often misleading as to a screenwriter's actual contribution to the finished product. On Beloved, *you are listed as one of three writers, coming after Akosua Busia and before Adam Brooks. What are we to make of that?*

Apparently the woman whose name came before mine had written a draft years before, but I had never read it.

Screenwriters define themselves in the industry by their credits. It must be frustrating when they don't accurately reflect who wrote what.

The WGA credit arbitration process is a difficult thing because they're judging creative work. Whether or not their formula works is up for discussion. Sometimes it does and sometimes it doesn't. I think sometimes it depends on who the arbitrators are. You never really know whether they're reading the material or not. You're not allowed to appeal your case. It's a very closed system. And they have a real sense of protection of the first writer. It's kind of the abused-child syndrome. They automatically assume that the first writer is being abused or taken advantage of, but that isn't always the case.

The problem is that there are a number of people who write who aren't screenwriters, but anybody can call themselves one. Everybody has their real job . . . and they're a screenwriter. I don't know why everybody thinks they can do it. So a dentist who decides he wants to adapt *Oliver Twist* can do that, it can be completely unfilmable and lacking in craft, but because he did the first version before someone else takes it and rewrites it, he could get a credit. That's just the way the system works.

Stephen Schiff, who wrote the scripts for *The Deep End of the Ocean* (1999) and *Lolita* (1997), makes a great argument on this subject, and he helped make some changes to the process.[2] Let's say that one writer does an adaptation of *Exodus* which doesn't work, and then a second writer comes in and makes it a script that can actually get made. Both writers are going to include the parting of the Red Sea, but do you credit the parting of the Red Sea to the first writer? No, because it was in *Exodus*. How much do you credit the first writer when he is working with ideas that already exist? Sometimes it's hard to judge.

You obviously read novels as they're offered to you for adaptation, but do you read a lot simply as a civilian?

I try to. I think too many screenwriters are referencing other screenplays, or other movies, as opposed to getting their source from the really good writing you find in novels. But I know that a lot of the really great screenwriters working today are really great readers. I know Tony Gilroy reads a lot, and Paul Thomas Anderson.

Are you able to read books simply for the enjoyment, or do you automatically start thinking about how you would adapt them?

I just enjoy them. It's like a vacation from the usual demands of my job.

Can you see yourself ever writing a novel?

My joke response is I don't know enough words. The most attractive part of writing a book is that you write without any kind of committee standing over you. You get to write what you want to write. I know you have an editor, but that's nothing compared to what a screenwriter has to go through. So just the experience of writing and having that creative experience being unimpeded by stop signs and notes and other people urinating on your territory would be a really great experience. You get to really see what you can do because you're creatively following you own muse without any other voices.

What was great in the '90s with screenwriters like Quentin Tarantino was that their writing and their style was more important to them than writing for the marketplace. They weren't writing for the industry and trying to get movie stars to do their scripts. Suddenly this whole crop of young, wonderful writers was working in an age where the writers were able to finance their films without having to go to the studios first and they could really see their own visions brought to the screen. Working in that environment, you become a better writer because you're making your own mistakes and finding your own successes. You're getting your own original voice out there.

My generation was right before that. I got into the studio system and was just so grateful to be working, but I am weaning myself away from that now.

It's hard to look at your list of produced credits and not see the remarkable number of films which are about and/or for women.

I was raised by women. I was surrounded by women. I had two older sisters, and my mom was one of four sisters. Because I was the only boy and because my father was kind of a distant figure in my early years because of his job as a cab driver—and because I wasn't the kind of boy he expected—I was very much in my mother's world. So when she would go visit her sisters, she'd take me along and I came to absorb women's voices all my life.

One of my sisters was seven years older than me and going through all the things that teenagers in the late '60s went through, and I was her confessor. She'd tell me everything. So as a little boy I heard all the stories about what she was going through. I just listened a lot. I wasn't a big talker in my family, I was pretty quiet. So I just absorbed a lot of female voices, sometimes to my own detriment as a man. Some of the things they said about men were things that I probably should never have heard as a little boy.

Such as?

Men are assholes, men are blowhards *[laughs]*. Many of the men in my family were not men who were able to support their families, so I heard a lot of the negative stuff. And a lot of the pain that women felt, because they loved their men anyway. There was still that kind of conflict.

Since you've had so much success writing for women, does that pigeonhole you in the industry?

To a certain extent, but I don't find it pigeonholing because it's in accord with my interests. But one of my favorite themes is male bonding. One of my favorite movies is *Gunga Din* (1939). I love movies about men who are just great friends and would die for each other. That's a theme I'm looking forward to exploring.

Do you have a regular writing routine that you've developed over the years?

After twenty years of doing this I finally have my own office. Before now I always had to work within other spaces. But I wake up, do my morning ablutions. I have a kind of meditation routine which I may do in the morning or at night depending on the energy of that day.

A lot of screenwriting is just showing up. You have to meet the page and see what happens. Sometimes you sit there musing and there are days and days with nothing happening, or what is happening is crap. And then you'll have one day a week where you're in the zone and hours go by and you make some sort of breakthrough. What's wonderful about this gig is that it's different all the time. But what's consistent is that you have to show up to write. You can't avoid it. And we writers do avoid it a lot. We clean, we go to book stores, we go to the movies, we go for a walk, we go to the gym. But if I'm working on something, sometimes I have my best ideas at the gym. I came up with most of the sequences in *Living Out Loud* when I was running at the gym. Sometimes you need to get away from the desk, or out from under your desk, to get your body moving so ideas can start rolling.

How big a part does research play in what you do?

In the beginning, I was not an enthusiastic researcher. It felt too much like homework, but I have really embraced it. It is so liberating. Research really fills up the well when you're dry.

When I was young, I thought, "Oh, I'm an artist. I should just create reality," which was all bullshit. I resisted it somewhat. Sometimes for me research was more about tone or feeling. For *A Little Princess,* I wanted to know more about India, so I did a ton of research about the period, what songs were popular, what were the major news events. And I watched *The Jewel in the Crown* (TV miniseries, 1984), which gave me a sense of the costumes and the set design.

What are the intangibles in your job which people might not know about?

I love collaboration. I get really excited sitting in a room with people I respect creatively and just jamming on ideas. Writing is such an isolated and introverted job. That's part of what's fun about directing is that you get to be more social and be with a group of people. If you're lucky enough to be with people you respect and who are smart, it's just fantastic.

My production designer on *P.S. I Love You* would bring me designs which would inspire me to write scenes a certain way. Or I'd go on a great location and think, "Wow, I wrote the scene like *this,* but now I see it that *this* would be even better." The thing that keeps me excited about the job is the excitement that comes from the evolution of the material once I start expanding beyond the room where I write. And I still have the dream of writing something truly great. I still don't think I've done that yet. I don't even know what form it will take, but it's that Don Quixote dream I have. That keeps me going.

April 2008

RICHARD LAGRAVENESE (1959–)

1989 *Rude Awakening* (David Greenwalt, Aaron Russo). Co-script.
1991 *The Fisher King* (Terry Gilliam). Script.
1994 *The Ref* (Ted Demme). Producer, co-script.
1995 *A Little Princess* (Alfonso Cuarón). Co-script.
The Bridges of Madison County (Clint Eastwood). Script.
Unstrung Heroes (Diane Keaton). Script.
1996 *The Mirror Has Two Faces* (Barbra Streisand). Script.
1998 *The Horse Whisperer* (Robert Redford). Co-script.
Living Out Loud (Richard LaGravenese). Director, script.
Beloved (Jonathan Demme). Co-script.
2003 *A Decade under the Influence* (Ted Demme, Richard LaGravenese). Producer, co-director (documentary film).
2006 *Paris, je t'aime* (segment "Pigalle") (Richard LaGravenese). Director, script.
2007 *Freedom Writers* (Richard LaGravenese). Director, script.
P.S. I Love You (Richard LaGravenese). Director, co-script.

Academy Award honors include a nomination for Best Original Screenplay for *The Fisher King*. Writers Guild honors also include a nomination for Best Original Screenplay for *The Fisher King*.

NOTES

1 Primarily a playwright, Alfred Uhry has won the Tony (twice), a Pulitzer Prize, and an Oscar, the latter for *Driving Miss Daisy* (1989). His infrequent screen credits include *Mystic Pizza* (1988).

2 In November 2002, the Writers Guild made a change to its arbitration rules in an attempt to ensure that the first writer on an adaptation did not receive undue credit for utilizing source material. The specific wording is: "Arbiters should give weight to any writer's original and unique utilization, choice, or arrangement of source material when it is present in the final shooting script, but not the employment of basic story elements which any other writer may have also selected."

INTERVIEW BY **PATRICK McGILLIGAN**

BARRY LEVINSON THE JOURNEY

Largely because of *Diner* (1982), *Tin Men* (1987), *Avalon* (1990), and *Liberty Heights* (1999), the engaging quartet of "Baltimore films" that explore his own life story and that of his friends and family, Barry Levinson looms as a towering figure among contemporary writer-directors. His chutzpah in making autobiographical films is as rare in mainstream Hollywood nowadays as it was in 1982, the year *Diner* was released, establishing Levinson, although he was a longtime veteran of the industry, as a new titan.

One year after turning auteur with *Diner,* Levinson made the decision to direct another writer's screenplay and resist any pigeonholing as a personal filmmaker. He also towers in his field as a "mere" director of films as intelligent as they are entertaining. *The Natural* (1984), *Good Morning, Vietnam* (1987), *Rain Man* (1988), *Bugsy* (1991), *Disclosure* (1994), *Wag the Dog* (1997), and *Sphere* (1998) are among the best known of his directorial (and nonwriting) hits. Indeed, though he has three Academy Award nominations for Best Script, his only Oscar is for directing *Rain Man.*

Writing, directing, and producing—not always doing all three at the same time—Levinson has amassed a long list of credits. Among contemporaries only Steven Spielberg seems as prolific. Occasionally, as with the compelling *Sleepers* (1996), Levinson adapts someone else's memoiristic fiction and evokes a world close to his own. And among his numerous credits are low-profile works destined to be rediscovered: I especially treasure *An Everlasting Piece* (2000), a barmy Irish comedy with a cast of eccentrics, none of them marquee names in America; and the picaresque, more all-star *Bandits* (2001). Both have all the humor, humanity, and quirky narrative structure of the "Baltimore films."

Lately, Levinson has gone back into television in a major way, writing, directing, and producing several acclaimed shows, the biggest attention-getters being *Oz*, an unflinching look at life inside a maximum security prison, and *Homicide: Life on the Streets*, a crime program set in his beloved Baltimore. He won an Emmy for Best Director in 1993 and three Peabodys for *Homicide* (1993, 1995, 1997).

Back, because, after graduating from college and landing his first television job in Washington, D.C., Levinson moved to Los Angeles and started out in local TV, writing and performing in a variety show, which led to network series with Marty Feldman, Tim Conway, and soon enough, Carol Burnett. He collected three Emmys as one of the team writing *The Carol Burnett Show*. He then found a most unlikely feature film mentor in Mel Brooks, and picked up the first of his Oscar nominations for Best Script as one of the collegial group responsible for *Silent Movie* (1976).

These days, at least half the time Levinson prefers to live in Connecticut and make his films and TV shows from his headquarters there, another way in which he resists pigeonholing.

. . .

What kind of film buff were you, growing up? Did you dream of making movies?

Look, I went to the movies every Saturday. That's what we did growing up. I always liked movies. And later, once we got cars and could drive, we used to go to an arthouse theater in Baltimore called the Playhouse. This was at the beginning of the French New Wave and Ingmar Bergman and Fellini. I used to see all the new foreign films there and I loved certain ones like the Ealing comedies. So I used to see a lot of films, but just as a kid, enjoying movies; I liked all these different types of films but I didn't see it as anything other than being a member of the audience. I was not watching films for style or technique, or taking the script apart.

What sort of writing did you do as a boy, growing up? Anything?

Mainly school papers, but I failed at everything I wrote. I was always in trouble with my school papers and therefore never thought I could actually write.

Were you writing badly, or out of the box?

I was writing, as it turns out, very outside of what the expectations were. For instance, I remember having to write a book report on *Catcher in the Rye*, and I wrote the book report mimicking the way Holden Caulfield spoke. So the book report began something like: "I really hate to write book reports, but if I do have to write a book report, then . . ." Basically adopting his voice. Then I'd get a failed grade because it wasn't any kind of conventional book report.

In college I was in broadcast journalism, but I took a course in creative writing, so somewhere in the back of my mind I must have liked the idea of writing, although I didn't really think much about it. That particular course, that professor, had a key, simple idea. When you wrote something, the professor read it to the class. Grades meant nothing to me; they made no difference. But I felt an obligation not to bore the class. So I wrote in a way intended to really engage the other students, and that was the first time I made the connection between writing and an audience.

Television was your real school of writing, wasn't it?

There were two great learning curves for me. One was working in local television in Washington, D.C., after college. I was in a training program to learn all the facets of television and you started out as what they called a "floor director." One of my early jobs was rolling in the commercial breaks between *The Late Show* and *The Late Late Show. The Late Show* began after the news, eleven-thirty P.M., and ran until, like, one-thirty A.M., and then the other movie would come on and run until three in the morning. I did that job for a time, rolling in the commercial breaks, and I began to see all these old movies that I wasn't even aware of. I'd just be sitting there, but you had to pay attention in order to roll in the breaks, so I began to watch all of these movies and suddenly notice things: "Oh, that's nice . . . that's well-done . . . interesting . . . who was that director?" I began to pay attention, not just being entertained like when I was younger. I began to pay attention to shots and lighting and directors. I began to recognize names like John Ford and Welles and Hawks. I began to have my own private education.

The other experience was being in acting school when I first came to Los Angeles. I didn't want to be an actor and I couldn't tell you what I was doing in an acting class, but I was fascinated by the class and I was fascinated by the class exercises. One of the things we used to do was improvisational exercises. I would do these improvisations and I found that, when I was improvising, I was able to come up with a lot of lines that were funny or interesting, et cetera. The reason those lines were coming out of my mouth is that I was playing a character, and I had a certain motivation, and therefore the lines came out naturally, rather than my thinking to myself, "What should I say here? What's a funny line here?" It only happened spontaneously based on my listening, and my reaction to the moment in terms of the character I was playing. Lines would come out. Behavior would speak. That is when I realized, "Oh! I don't even have to do improvisation. I can simply write it down, as long as I allow the same mindset to work." Like, "I'm walking into a room at a party, I feel awkward . . . Okay, now that I'm in that particular environment, now that I'm in that moment, what do I say, how do I behave?" Then the lines would begin to come out on the page, not only my lines, but whoever else I was playing. When I began to play all the characters in my head, the characters began to interact with one another.

So improvisation became your bridge to writing.

It was the key element. Because otherwise all you're trying to do is say lines without the focus that comes from the acting exercises. Improvisation contributed to my ability to write characters. It was the key, because now you are stepping into the character and you become the person, you become all the characters. When you become them, you begin to understand how they think and what their motivation is; they begin to speak and come alive.

• • •

What was your first professional writing job?

Eventually I got a job working on a local television show in Los Angeles called *The Lohman and Barkley Show.* It was originally a ninety-minute weekend show, done live on tape; you did it live and they taped it for playback a few hours later. We came in on Monday mornings and by Friday we needed to have ninety minutes of material. It was like *Saturday Night Live* before *Saturday Night Live.*

Didn't you have to show them some writing in order to get the job?

Generally you would, but by the fluke of it I had met with the producers and we talked, and they took a liking to me, along with Craig T. Nelson, who had been in my same acting class. The two of us were playing clubs together. Craig and I both ended up getting hired to write and perform for this show.

You took it to another level, writing for national network television series and for comedians like Tim Conway and Marty Feldman, and ultimately for The Carol Burnett Show. *Writing for such shows gets complicated, doesn't it? You have to think of yourself as Carol Burnett's alter ego, playing the characters.*

Now I was writing sketches, and sketches are like minimovies. You have to have a setup, a plot, and a conclusion. You have to come up with an idea that allows for a character to be funny. Just to give you an example: We'd come into work and be talking about Dr. Jekyll and Mr. Hyde, and someone would say—because this was the era of women's lib—"Why don't we do Dr. Jekyll and Ms. Hyde? Harvey Korman is working on a potion, and he turns into Carol . . . ; the transformation will be hilarious." So we have our premise for a five-minute sketch, we know how Harvey and Carol will function within the piece, and you just know they both will work it and sell it.

What made Carol so great, for a writer, was she didn't just read cue cards like a lot of variety show people were doing. She became the characters. For example, you could imagine a quiet woman working in an office . . . get inside that character's head. You could write wonderful moments, marvelous characters, and Carol could inhabit them.

Of course sketches were sketches, and I became tired of sketches and that's what led to screenwriting.

You were taken under wing by Mel Brooks, as one of his comedy writers. Is there a way you can characterize what Mel contributed to your growth as a writer?

A lot of things. In many ways, I was lucky to work with Mel, me and my partner at the time—Rudy DeLuca—and Rod Clark. We would meet with Mel for breakfast, fool around and talk—talk about scenes and other stuff—and then go to the office and write; we'd go to lunch, talk some more, and do more writing in the afternoon. We spent a long time doing just that. Not only did we help write the scripts, Mel included us when he was casting, locations, filming—and then ultimately all the way through the editing process. It truly was what you might call an apprenticeship. I was exposed to everything about the making of the film, from the script all the way through to completion. So you saw how some ideas that were wonderful didn't translate; you saw how certain great moments somehow never materialized on camera, and how moments that weren't quite as good on paper became better on film. You saw the whole fragility of the process, how delicate it all is, from beginning to end. That was an invaluable three years of my life.

I don't think most people think of you as in any way connected with that kind of low, vaudeville, bad-taste comedy [laughs]. *I mean, I love Mel's films, so I say that appreciatively, but I think of you as more of a humanist interested in character-driven stories. Is there any way you can isolate your function within that group?*

There are different ways you can function as a writer. But one way is you can inhabit a particular sensibility, and play it out. You step into that sensibility. You can see it with comedians who have a completely different persona offstage, because they are always playing a character. The same thing applies to writing at times. It doesn't mean it's your favorite form or your first love, but you can do that.

In group writing like that, was it partly a game of topping one another?

No, I don't think it was competitive. There was a joy in the group. Mel would say something and you'd laugh your head off, then someone else would say something and we'd laugh harder, and Mel would say, "Put that down. Let's use that!" Mel was obviously the leader—it was a Mel Brooks movie after all and you were only a contributor—but you cannot feel inhibited, or you won't say anything.

It seems to me you were moving gradually from improvisation to sketch material to group writing, eventually down to partnering with your then-wife, Valerie Curtin, all of it on the way, subconsciously or otherwise, towards writing alone. After writing with your wife you don't ever again collaborate with a regular writing partner. You go solo and stay solo.

Eventually you want to do a work based on one voice. It happened with *Diner*, and, oddly enough, it was Mel who was probably the most encouraging in that regard. We spent so many hours sitting and talking, and we'd talk about all sorts of things. I used to tell stories about what I referred to as "the diner guys," and Mel used to say, "You should write about that," and I'd say, "Yeah, but I don't know what the story is." He told me to watch Fellini's movie *I vitelloni* (1953) and think about it. Time would pass, and he'd ask "What are you doing with 'the diner guys'? You should do something!" I couldn't get my head wrapped around the idea until I realized it wasn't only about the guys, but about the fact that we were so close because of our fear of female relationships and our lack of understanding of women.

And it took several years of talking and thinking about it?

It just rolled around in my head during that time. All of a sudden, one day, I went, "Oh! Oh! Okay!" All of a sudden, bang. Everything made sense. Until then, I had all these little stories in my head but not something that would push me to start writing.

Diner *was the first of the true "Baltimore films." But I've read somewhere that you consider . . .* And Justice for All *and* Best of Friends *to be Baltimore films that had to be more commercial, as well as directed by other people, because of the phase of your career you were in.*

Yeah, I think that's true. . . . *And Justice for All* came about because one of my friends, one of the diner guys, became a lawyer, and whenever I went back to Baltimore he would tell me these stories about what was going on in the legal system and how screwed up it all was. He told me these completely crazy stories. I used to tell his stories to Valerie, and eventually that evolved into . . . *And Justice for All.* It was all based on the diner guy who became a lawyer and that whole legal world in Baltimore. If I hadn't done . . . *And Justice for All* earlier, it would have been one of the Baltimore pieces after *Diner* and *Tin Men.* It would have been a little differently structured, done in a different fashion, but certainly connected.

But preceding Diner, Best of Friends *was your first truly autobiographical script, not about one of your friends, but about you and your life and your marriage and your collaboration.*

Yes, that was really about Valerie and me and the time we were together, getting married and visiting our folks, and our lives as writers.

Writing with a partner is in some ways an easy but odd process. Two people come into a room and look to each other for motivation. One might not be in the right mood at any given moment. And somehow you begin, somehow, out of your exchanges of thoughts, something engages both of you, and the process of collaboration begins. But sometimes it's a struggle to focus two minds in a single direction. That's not to say a writing partnership can't be exciting and unpredictable in good ways, but you're both filtering ideas through one another, and sometimes the energies are different, and there are a lot of bumpy moments.

Best of Friends *is set in a commercial framework, though—so that the audience doesn't really have to know it is autobiographical.*

No, it plays as a romantic comedy.

. . .

I read somewhere that when you finally wrote Diner, *the words practically gushed out, that you dictated the script to a secretary and it was all written very quickly. Is that true?*

I did write it quickly. I wrote it in three weeks, but I write all of the Baltimore pieces easily and quickly. They come out in about a three-week period. I didn't dictate *Diner,* but I did dictate a few of the others.

How are you able to do that, dictate? Does it come out of your improvisational background, the ability to pace and think and get into the characters and speak the lines?

Yes, exactly.

I would have thought the Baltimore films would be harder to write. Or more emotionally taxing.

They're complicated, very complicated. *Avalon* was extremely complicated in its form.

But you still crank them out in three weeks?

They come out very quickly once they are ready to come out.

Are they researched beforehand? I know you don't have to research what you might distinctly remember, but on the other hand not everything is always remembered clearly. And I read in your novel Sixty-six *that you wonder sometimes if what you remember, especially the stories that overlap other people's, is your memory, or a kind of collective memory.*

I did this much for *Avalon:* I went back to Baltimore and I spoke to members of the family that were still around and I collected pieces of information. I spent a few weeks in Baltimore, just talking to family members.

That's the only time you did that? Not with Diner? *You didn't go back and talk to the diner guys?*

No.

Were you, as time passed, and you were letting the ideas roll around inside your head, making notes and dropping them into a box labeled "The Diner Guys Movie"?

No. I had no notes.

You started without notes? It was all in your head?

Right.

What did you know starting out, the beginning and the end?

That's a good question. I have an idea how it's going to end. It's almost like looking through this long tube and you can see all the way down to the end but you don't know exactly what's along the way. What I had to do is go back to the improvisational exercises that I did in acting class, and I had to trust myself, and that's a big order.

As a writer you understand, at the beginning, that you have structural commitments to a screenplay. You know you will need certain elements along the way that will engage an audience. You have to keep them committed to the film. Then you have to put those things away in the back of your head, and you have to trust that the characters are going to be alive enough that they will ultimately push you in ways that you're not necessarily aware of, starting out; the characters will change the boundaries, even, of what you have laid out in your own head. Sometimes they will say things that are unexpected, and sometimes their behavior will go beyond what you had thought they would do.

You have to move ahead without trepidation, without being fearful of some calamity that you're thrusting upon yourself. You have to trust that somehow you're going to get through this journey, and that the writing will be at times seemingly almost spontaneous, because it's behavior, while at the same time that the script will never go off into left field without making sense in terms of the overall structure.

All this time it's simply in your head? You don't have any treatment on the desk in front of you. . . ?

I don't know how to write a treatment.

Or a step outline?

I don't know how to do any of those things.

Is that true of all your scripts, not just the Baltimore films?

That's true about most things I write, although some things, just by their nature, will be different.

Is the pipeline of Baltimore films endless? Because I know that now you have switched to writing those memories as fiction, putting those kinds of stories into your first novel, Sixty-six, *and that worries me.*

I think *Sixty-six* is probably the last one. If I make *Sixty-six* into a movie, that will be the end of them.

Really? That's a pretty momentous decision. Why? Because it's such a struggle to convince the studios that there's money in such films nowadays?

Yeah. Times ultimately change. The economics of trying to do a period movie have become more complicated, a lot more complicated. Films that are personal as well as period are more and more difficult to do. If you look at the realities, there's a cutoff point where you're not going to get that type of project through anymore. I look at *Sixty-six* as the conclusion, because in my head that was the end of the *Diner* era, the breakup of the guys, and when I went west. So it's a natural conclusion for me.

Although it seems to me, off the top of my head, that you spent so much interesting time in television—that you could continue into television, L.A., and the early 1960s. Of course, then, it wouldn't be a Baltimore film, except for your character coming from Baltimore.

You're right, I could continue. There's a great story in some of the experiences I first had in L.A. and they might be humorous and dramatic in the same way as the Baltimore pieces. But I think there gets to be a point in time, with the corporatization of film, that personal filmmaking really isn't feasible.

. . .

Starting with The Natural *in 1984, you've directed a lot of other people's scripts. Being a writer, originally, when you are directing a script written by someone else, where you don't intend to take any writing credit, how do you go about asking for rewrites, or editing or tinkering with the script? It must be difficult for a younger writer to approach you for your opinion.*

Basically you talk it over. You don't say, "Go rewrite it and come back." You talk about it, and through the conversations and discussions certain things become more clear. I don't try to impose myself as a writer, in that way. There are ways to work with a writer in which you can evolve a script or enhance it in subtle ways that sometimes have a very strong effect.

When you started out directing other people's scripts, was that philosophy of working with a writer as a director a learning process for you? Or did it come about more naturally as a result of having come in under all those group-writing experiences?

Collaborating with others for so many years, I did learn there are ways to accomplish what you are after by nurturing the creative flow. I try not to impose my personality over someone else's to the extent that I inhibit them. You need to be open and explore, while heading where you want to go.

You can never be too in love with your own ideas. If you can remember every idea that is yours in a script, as opposed to someone else's, then something is wrong. Like when I was working with Mel, I honestly can't remember who thought up this idea or that idea in particular scenes, it was usually a group effort. It was really a collaboration.

*Looking at it in terms of famous examples from your career—*Good Morning, Vietnam; Rain Man; Bugsy; and Wag the Dog*—from the outside looking in, one might think those were perfect scripts and all you had to do—a tall order, regardless—was say, "Great, let's go to work and film it." Are there times when you are obliged to do a little writing?*

It's funny, but you mention *Good Morning, Vietnam* and *Rain Man.* Both of those were problematic scripts. I don't think you would have filmed those scripts as is, because they needed a lot of elements to make the movie come to life, in a way that was slightly unpredictable at the outset. It's very seldom you can take a script and just shoot it. But those two needed to be enhanced.

Tell me about Good Morning, Vietnam. *Was it changed during filming partly because of Robin Williams?*

Yes. You want to take advantage of his comedic mind. Use it. His full personality hadn't been fully realized in his earlier films. In the case of *Good Morning, Vietnam* it would have been foolish not to find or bring to the screen a mind like no other I had come across before. That applied also to the Vietnamese, who couldn't do the lines as written. In read-throughs and rehearsals, I could see they were saying lines they couldn't handle. That stuff in the classroom scenes, for example, didn't work. It sounded like lines.

So then you start making changes. You talk to them and find out what they'd really say. Finally you get to a point where you say, "The hell with it. Let's not even slate the scene. We'll tail-slate it, and just let Robin talk, and let the other actors respond to Robin."

All those scenes became improvised. For the first time you began to hear the Vietnamese speaking in a way that was natural and not simply spewing out lines. The sequences got built without anybody knowing we were filming. In that way you get the behavior of the people in the classroom that is much closer to what they are really about, rather than lines on a piece of paper they can't quite deliver. I don't do that out of disregard for the screenwriter; it's a matter of taking a look at what's happening in a given moment and saying, "We're not going to get there if we go down this road, so I have to make course corrections." I had to build those scenes between Robin and the Vietnamese in a way that seemed more naturalistic and lively and more credible.

It seems you have a policy of never taking credit on a script that you are directing, which someone else wrote.

Right.

So that whatever you might do to enhance the script, you are not standing in front of the writer.

Right.

Alfred Hitchcock had a similar philosophy. He wrote or helped write all of his movies, yet there came a point in his career when he stopped taking any script credit. The possessory credit covered it all for him.

Right. That's very true. And look, no matter what, it starts with the writer. The writer has put something on the page and that's what you ultimately are committed to filming. Whatever course corrections need to be made, or adjustments that pop up, it still began with the writer.

In terms of *Rain Man* there was a writer's strike, and so I went off with the script I had at that time, and things happened on the road and changes were made because of what happened on the road. The script evolved.

Again, the writer wasn't with you?

No.

So you had to do a little writing and some fixes?

Because of the nature of the piece. If you're making a movie about an autistic, you have a choice. You can do a tightly constructed piece, but making it so tightly constructed you'll knock out some of the behavioral aspects of the two main characters. My feeling grew on the road that the behavior and the relationship were the most interesting aspects of the piece, not the plot points that were supposedly to be followed. Because autism was an affliction that few people had heard of at that time, few people understood it, and we didn't want to explain it in great detail. I wanted to show how the behavior works, and that is the way the audience would understand it. I wanted to show the frustrations of someone who deals with an autistic, and also the frustrations of the autistic himself, who is kind of locked in a mental box, and then we wanted to show this behavior unfold as the two guys go from Cincinnati to Los Angeles.

You had to be open enough to see little things happen, and then build on them. On the road we kept building. For example, Dustin [Hoffman] came up to me one day and said something like, "I have this business I do when I get agitated. I go into this pitching motion, this long, slow windup. Only it takes too much time, I think. I wish there was something else I could do that took less time." I said, "Try 'Who's on first?'" He said, "Who do you mean 'Who's on first?'" I said, "The Abbott and Costello routine." He said, "Who's playing the other guy?" I said, "You do both and do it like a mantra. You speak the words but you don't understand the humor, because you're an autistic. It's a rhythm that you're into, a mantra, that can alleviate your frustration." He said, "That's interesting." I checked with some psychologists who understand autism, and they said it was plausible. And that's how that got into the movie.

Later on, I figured out Dustin's character would get agitated by the mantra at times, because at a certain point things like that can drive you crazy. And then we could have Tom [Cruise] getting angry, saying, "Don't you understand? That's a joke! It's a comedy routine!" So "Who's on first?" ran all the way through the movie. Things like that happen as you go along, if you're open enough.

Another example: One day I got worried that the audience would think Tom wasn't taking good enough care of Dustin, and that led me to the underwear-at-K-Mart bit. Tom saying, "What about your underwear? I gave you underwear . . ." Dustin saying, "I only get my underwear at K-Mart in Cincinnati." We were trying to show how the rigidity of the rituals of autism plays out, in a natural way. That was another sequence that evolved when we were on the road. All those things got added along the journey; you observe the behavior and the relationships, and you take advantage. We built on things as we followed the characters on the journey, cross-country.

What about Bugsy?

Bugsy was a different process. Warren approached me with Jimmy Toback's screenplay. It was probably 200 to 250 pages, with some incredible stuff in it. We moved forward to make the movie. Warren, Jimmy, and I would meet constantly and work on aspects of it, talk about ideas, how we could embellish certain things. It was an ongoing process all through preproduction, even into the shooting. It was one of the great collaborations in that regard.

Was it different with Wag the Dog? *Because David Mamet is such a precise, lapidary writer?*

He's fantastic, but even so, some improvisational stuff just creeps in. Sometimes, because of the dynamic of that group, things happened. Other times, it's exactly the way David wrote it.

Each script that you do—between the writer, the actors, the director, and the environment that you're in—these will determine how the scenes will play out.

. . .

Starting out as a writer, did you ever read or study a classic film script?

Never saw one. Didn't even know how to write a script, until I actually wrote my first one, sometime in the late 1960s, and then I had to buy a book that told you how to do the format. You know: INTERIOR. BEDROOM. DAY. CUT TO . . . I had to have a book about the format because I didn't know anything about it.

Is that the first script you wrote from beginning to end?

That's the first I started from scratch.

What was it about? Did it ever get made?

No, it never did. I just wrote it. To be honest with you, I haven't looked at it in thirty years, but it was about what we were discussing—my journey into Los Angeles and the beginning of my living in L.A.

So it was autobiographical but relatively contemporaneous with your life at the time.

Yes.

Do you remember the circumstances under which you wrote it? Because things have changed so much for screenwriters over recent years, even the physical ways of doing the work. Were you using a typewriter, pencil and paper, working at home or the office?

The way I normally used to write was in longhand, and then I'd type it up shortly after I had written *x* number of pages, because if I stayed away from the pages for too long I wouldn't be able to read my own handwriting. I wrote so fast and so sloppy. I'd go from yellow pages to typing pages, then go back and write some more on yellow pages. But everything I wrote was all in longhand.

Everything was so laborious in those days, even the typewriters and the script formatting.

A major pain. You had to take your script to a place that put it into the proper format and then to another place to get it printed, and that all took three days. If there were any mistakes or revisions, you had to do it all over again.

Has the format changed drastically for you, from those days? Did some of the formatting become old-fashioned?

Scripts are a little less formal. I think William Goldman might have been the first to break certain conventions. I remember reading *Butch Cassidy and the Sundance Kid* (1969), and he'd write something like, "Then Butch gives him the greatest kick in the balls in cinematic history." Or the phrase you hear throughout the movie, "Who are those guys?"—he was filling you in differently than in the past. That was not how a script was normally written in the past.

Plus he put in less camerawork or camera instructions.

Yes.

Has your own style changed?

The way I wrote is pretty much the way that I write. I never used to describe things in great detail. I was always fairly sparse.

So your scripts were and are dialogue-focused.

Yes. If you think of *Diner,* it was dialogue-focused. I think it wasn't difficult to read but it was easy to misunderstand. I remember the initial reaction from agents. "I don't know, there's not much here . . . " Once you talked them through it, explaining the characters, they'd say, "Oh I see!" Because there weren't people commenting throughout on what good friends the characters were.

People actually had to read the script diligently and finish it.

Yes.

Characters' names are so important. Do you have any tricks for coming up with them?

No, no tricks. Sometimes I write in the names of people that I knew, in some cases it's a name with a certain color. The names have to stick. If you keep changing them, that's a bad sign.

Has wearing so many hats—writing, directing, and producing (you do so much directing and producing nowadays, not to mention major activity in television)—has all this productivity in other areas hindered your writing? I mean, has there been any downside to your writing, stemming from that productivity as a director and producer? I would imagine that nowadays you don't always have the time to write, or to develop that intimacy with the material.

No, because at the end of the day it's all about an intimacy with the material. At some point, it's only about that. You can't just simply say, "OK, what do we have to shoot today, three pages?" It goes way beyond that. You've been living with the characters in your head all the way from the first reading to the whole preproduction period, including looking at the locations. Because sometimes you go to a location and you realize, "Oh my god, we're going to have to make changes in this particular scene because it isn't going to quite work." Or: "This can be even stronger than I imagined." Little adjustments are happening all the time. All along you're making decisions about how the film will evolve, the problems there are in a scene, things that might have to be added because of a lack of clarity in a certain moment. The way I work, the only way I know how to work, is that once you are basically committed to go ahead with a project, the script—the scenes, the characters—are running around in your head all the time.

Yet there seems to be quite a gap of time between Liberty Heights *and* Man of the Year, *as though you made a conscious decision to write less, and direct and produce more. As you shifted into television, and more directing and producing, you must have borrowed the time away from writing. From your point of view, it doesn't really take you away from writing?*

Maybe, but there's a period of time when you're just not interested in certain things and your motivation is not the same.

Are you saying this was a period of time when you weren't as interested in writing and your motivations for writing had changed in the last several years?

Certain ideas aren't pushing you the same. Certain ideas come up to you and start pushing you. Sometimes it doesn't happen that way, so you have to just let things be. I don't want to feel as though I have to run out and write something all the time. I wait until it gets under my skin, and then I've just got to do it.

Do you search for something to write? Do you look for ways to refresh your writer's creativity, or do you just wait for that idea to come along and nudge you?

I wait for something to nudge me. Suddenly things start to speak to you. I don't know that you can generate it.

You don't have some ritual vacation that you take between films in order to do nothing but walk up and down on the beach, soul-searching. You don't feel antsy about writing?

I don't, unless something is percolating and then I let my instincts take over rather than push it.

Is living and working in Connecticut part of the time intended to give you a real as well as psychological distance from Hollywood?

I think so. People say a lot of silly things about Los Angeles. It's a place which has good and bad things about it, like everywhere else. For me, the big thing is I get tired of everyone talking about the business all the time. I yearn to go for breakfast some place like here, sit with a paper and read and hang out for an hour; some place where I'm not going to be sitting around talking about this or that film, or whatever. The time away from the business feels more like a life to me. But I don't have any anti-Hollywood sensibility.

What is the ideal writing situation for you nowadays? Where, for example, did you write Man of the Year*?*

I'm always in the house or where there are other things going on, when I'm writing. I know people think about Hemingway, off some place, sharpening his pencils before he heads for the typewriter, and there's something romantic about that image. But I find myself in any particular place where I can take note pads and start to work, generally close to where some music is playing, because I do play music all the time when I write.

Time of day?

Generally, when I'm writing, this is my schedule. I'll go out and have breakfast, read the paper and do some errands, come back, sit down, start to write. Write until lunch, take a break, then write until five-thirty in the evening.

Do you ever stare at the blank page and nothing comes?

No, I don't work that way. When I'm in the writing mode but the page is blank, I'm going through songs—just playing music.

Any particular type of music? Is it always '60s rock?

No. It depends on what I'm thinking about. I could be all over the place.

Jazz or classical?

I don't listen to that much jazz. Some, but not on a regular basis. Sometimes I'll get fixated on certain music for a certain script. I now notice, with the advent of iTunes, how many times I've played a given song. I'll see I played something 135 times while writing a particular script. When I did *Diner,* for example, I listened to Pete Townshend—that album *Empty Glass* with the song called "Rough Boys"—the entire time. And in those days the songs didn't just repeat; you had to get up, go over to the record machine, and put the needle down again.

So in a sense, music is your mantra—a trick not unlike Hemingway sharpening his pencils—letting your mind roam as you begin to write.

Yes.

You must get so much to read—what people send to you, what you come across in a bookstore, or what crosses your path on any given day. Do you read at all purely for pleasure, or to let your mind roam, without worrying about whether it might be suitable for a film?

More often than not I read biographies and nonfiction, if I'm reading just for pleasure.

What are you reading now, for example?

I've been reading a bunch of political books like *State of Denial,* Bob Woodward's book. I've been reading these books and thinking, if you were to look back at where we are one hundred years from now in the future, how would you view this time? In Woodward's book and a couple of others you see the behavioral aspects of the government in close-up, but I wonder how the overview will look different from the day-to-day intricacies. I've been intrigued by that premise. In the greater scheme it's an astounding tragedy that we are in the midst of, in America. To me, it's almost as though the country is involved in a coup, but we don't quite perceive it that way yet. Looking back, I wonder what the grand overview will be.

Are you saying you've been reading these books and involuntarily thinking of them as a film?

Involuntarily things keep popping in your head, but that doesn't mean you'll do anything about it.

That would be an interesting frame for a science-fiction film, looking back on this era from the future.

That's been in my head, but at the same time I'm just reading. When you're reading, things begin to stick. Not that you'll do anything with any of it. But it's the nature of being a writer. One of the things about being a writer is you have to be inquisitive and open to things that wander around and rattle in your head. Information keeps coming in and it creates internal scenarios.

One last question, a kind of trick question. I remember asking the same question of Julius J. Epstein once. I asked, was there a common thread to his many, many disparate films? He answered, "I always say, 'No man is an island,' because you can't refute it—and it works for everything." I know you pride yourself on the surprising variety of your work, but is there a common thread in what interests you as a writer and what interests you as a director or producer? A common idea? Does it always have to be something that resonates with you?

Yes, you have to find something that resonates, but you don't have to consciously be aware of it. If you look at any career, if you want to sit down and analyze a career, you can probably find all kinds of things that are there consistently. You can see the pathology of it all, but the pathology of it isn't that interesting to me, as opposed, simply, to the doing of it. Maybe later you can make some sense out of the resonance or the pathology, but I don't think these are necessarily things to keep in mind while you are doing it.

As a matter of fact, at least it seems to me, you try very hard to keep those things out of mind.

Yes, I do. I do!

September 2007

BARRY LEVINSON (1942–)

1975 *Street Girls* (Michael Miller). Co-script.
1976 *Silent Movie* (Mel Brooks). Co-script, actor.
1977 *High Anxiety* (Mel Brooks). Co-script, actor.
1979 *. . . And Justice for All* (Norman Jewison). Co-script.
1980 *Inside Moves* (Richard Donner). Co-script.

1981 *History of the World, Part 1* (Mel Brooks). Actor.

1982 *Diner* (Barry Levinson). Director, script.

Best Friends (Norman Jewison). Co-script.

Tootsie (Sydney Pollack). Uncredited contribution.

1984 *Unfaithfully Yours* (Howard Zieff). Script.

The Natural (Barry Levinson). Director.

1985 *Young Sherlock Holmes* (Barry Levinson). Director.

1987 *Tin Men* (Barry Levinson). Director, script.

Good Morning, Vietnam (Barry Levinson). Director.

1988 *Rain Man* (Barry Levinson). Director.

1990 *Avalon* (Barry Levinson). Producer, director, script.

1991 *Bugsy* (Barry Levinson). Producer, director.

Kafka (Steven Soderbergh). Executive producer.

1992 *Toys* (Barry Levinson). Producer, director, script.

1994 *Jimmy Hollywood* (Barry Levinson). Producer, director, script, actor.

Disclosure (Barry Levinson). Producer, director.

Quiz Show (Robert Redford). Actor.

1996 *Sleepers* (Barry Levinson). Producer, director, script.

1997 *Wag the Dog* (Barry Levinson). Producer, director.

Donnie Brasco (Mike Newell). Producer.

1998 *Sphere* (Barry Levinson). Producer, director.

Home Fries (Dean Parisot). Producer.

1999 *Liberty Heights* (Barry Levinson). Producer, director, script.

Original Diner Guys (Barry Levinson). Documentary film.

2000 *An Everlasting Piece* (Barry Levinson). Producer, director.

The Perfect Storm (Wolfgang Petersen). Executive producer.

2001 *Bandits* (Barry Levinson). Producer, director.

2002 *Possession* (Neil LaBute). Producer.

Analyze That (Harold Ramis). Executive producer.

2003 *Deliver Us from Eva* (Gary Hardwick). Executive producer.

2004 *Envy* (Barry Levinson). Producer, director.

2006 *Man of the Year* (Barry Levinson). Producer, director, script.

2008 *What Just Happened?* (Barry Levinson). Director.

2009 *Poliwood* (Barry Levinson). Director (documentary).

Published works include *Sixty-six: A Novel* (2003).

Television includes *The Lohman and Barkley Show* (1969 local Los Angeles series); *The Carol Burnett Show* (1969–70 series); *The Tim Conway Show* (1970 series); *The Marty Feldman Comedy Machine* (1971 series); "Diner" (1983 pilot for unproduced series); *The 20th Century: Yesterday's Tomorrows* (executive producer of 1999 documentary *Homicide: Life on the Street* (producer, director, and writer for 1993–99 series); *Oz* (executive producer of 1997 series); *The Second Civil War* (executive producer of 1997 telefilm); *Homicide: The Movie* (executive producer of 2000 telefilm); *American Tragedy* (executive producer of 2000 telefilm); *The Beat* (executive producer and director for the 2000 series); *Falcone* (executive producer of 2000 series); *Shot in the Heart* (executive producer of 2001 telefilm); *Hudson's Law* (executive producer of 2001 series); *Strip Search* (executive producer for 2004 telefilm); *The Jury* (executive producer, director, and writer for the 2004 series); *3 lbs.* (2005 pilot episode); *The Bedford Diaries* (executive producer of 2006 series); *M.O.N.Y.* (executive producer, director, and writer for the 2007 series).

"Webisodes" include *American Express Webisodes: The Adventures of Superman and Seinfeld* (two four-minute webisodes: "A Uniform Used to Mean Something" and "Hindsight is 20/20," directed by Levinson, 2004).

Academy Award honors include Best Original Script nominations for *... And Justice for All*, *Diner*, and *Avalon*. Levinson was nominated as Best Director for *Bugsy* (which was also nominated for Best Picture) and *Rain Man*, winning the directing Oscar for the latter. (*Rain Man* also earned the top directing award that year from the Directors Guild of America.)

Writers Guild honors include Best Original Script nominations for *Silent Movie* and *Diner*. He won the WGA's Best Script award for *Avalon*.

INTERVIEW BY **PATRICK McGILLIGAN**

ERIC ROTH PRIDE OF AUTHORSHIP

For the first two decades of his unorthodox career Eric Roth flew under the radar, leading a Forrest Gump–like seemingly ubiquitous existence behind the scenes. If he wasn't quite on the A-list in the 1970s, he circulated widely and made friends easily, building bridges to a future that would mark him as one of the screenwriting pantheon. At least Hollywood knew his name, and the literary quality of his work, even if that wasn't always reflected in the credits.

In 1994 he proved himself once and for all on *Forrest Gump*, the story of a lovable idiot that was also the story of turbulent America in the 1960s. People were swept away by the film: Tom Hanks's winning, star-making performance, the emotional sweep and crazy-quilt tapestry of the script, the quotable dialogue and memorable scenes, a soundtrack that couldn't be beat. *Gump* was a box-office phenomenon that year, and Roth won the Oscar for Best Screenplay.

Not an easy writer to pigeonhole, Roth then switched to serious, challenging, reality-based dramas like *The Insider* (1999) and *Ali* (2001), both directed by Michael Mann; *Munich* (2005), directed by Steven Spielberg; and *The Good Shepherd* (2006), with actor Robert De Niro directing the film as well as playing a role on-screen. Roth's collaborations on *The Insider* (with Mann) and *Munich* (with Pulitzer Prize–winning playwright Tony Kushner) also drew Academy Award nominations.

Born in New York, Roth was educated at the University of Santa Barbara (with graduate school stints at Columbia and UCLA). Adaptations of preexisting material are his specialty, but his long filmography is varied, and he continues to be amazingly productive. The full list of his work would include, besides his well-known scripts for Hollywood's best directors, all the times he has rewritten—and still rewrites—high-profile scripts, uncredited.

. . .

I'm interested in the fact that probably your first screen credit was on a documentary about the Poor People's Campaign.

The documentary was called *I Am Somebody*; that line was from a twenty-two-year-old—or whatever age he was—Jesse Jackson. Martin Luther King had planned a march on Washington for poor people, then he was assassinated, but organizers continued with planning for the march. Buses were going to D.C. from all over the country—"Watts to Washington" was the one we were with. As you went to each city you picked up another bus full of people so there was a whole caravan. It was a pretty interesting experience, not the happiest, but interesting.

You were on the bus with film equipment?

We had put together a group of about six of us. We each went on different buses, starting from different places. Everybody was going to what was called Resurrection City, a big tent city on the mall in Washington. When we got there we filmed inside the tent city and then went to the demonstrations taking place every day at various government buildings.

Did the documentary ever get shown?

It was shown a lot as fundraisers for like the Southern Christian Leadership Conference or the NAACP. It's a pretty good movie. I'm credited as one of the directors.

I know you went to graduate school first at Columbia and then UCLA. Did either of those schools give you the kind of connections to the film industry, which they are expected to do nowadays?

When I was at UCLA, I entered the Samuel Goldwyn writing contest, and I won that contest with a screenplay. Actually I tied with Colin Higgins, who went on to make *Harold and Maude* (1971), *9 to 5* (1980), and other films. *Harold and Maude* was the script that he wrote for the competition, his award-winning script. Anyway, we were joint winners, and that got me an agent, which was the most important thing that had happened in my career up to that time.

Was your script that won the Goldwyn prize ever filmed?

No. It was a fictional journey about a real-life incident involving Jerry Rubin, the politico. I was interested in Rubin, and what I was mostly interested in was that he had been in jail in Santa Rosa, California—for disturbing the peace or something—at the time he was indicted for the Chicago Conspiracy. So the government had to move him across the country for his trial, and they were afraid to put him on an airplane—which was ludicrous, but a true story—so they put him in a car with two FBI agents and a guy who was being extradited for murder, and drove cross-country. I thought that was a pretty intriguing idea for a movie, and that's what I wrote.

Nothing ever happened with it, but because of the prize a few agencies came to me, and I said I'd sign with whichever one could get me work—because I really wanted and needed work. A woman with a small agency came up with a job on a small oddball film that actually got made in Israel.

That's To Catch A Pebble. *What is that film about? Because you can't really see it nowadays.*

I don't know if you ever could see it *[laughs]*. My new agent sent me to an interesting, very nice man named Jim Collier, who was a big Christian and a filmmaker for Billy Graham's organization. He made somewhat religious films about subjects like the Holy Land. They were all fairly well-made films. He had an idea he wanted me to write into a script, and it was a paying job. It was a lay film, a love story, nothing religious about it, but it was set in Israel. The company that financed it was a travel company that sent tours to the Holy Land.

So I wrote the screenplay and got paid for it, which was great: my first professional job as a writer. Then they shot it in Israel, and we had a lot of fun going there. It was a small little tiny movie; the only name in the cast that anybody would recognize nowadays was a woman named Joanna Pettet, who was also in *The Group* and who was a kind of semistar in those days.

It never got much release in America?

Nah. I think it wasn't such a bad movie, though. The story was about a stewardess who had a relationship that was going bad and who decides not to return to America. She stays in Israel, trying to escape her bad relationship. She becomes involved with this young Israeli who takes her to the kibbutz where he grew up to meet his family. He's a sort of charming longhair, but it turns out the stewardess is pregnant by her old boyfriend, who then shows up.

Obviously it was a great experience being in Israel in 1969, but the best thing about the whole movie was the actor who played Joanna Pettet's American love interest, a man named William Jordan, who had a close relationship with the great playwright Lanford Wilson, who wrote *Hot L*

Baltimore and *Talley's Folley.* Lanford Wilson came over to Israel and actually helped me write one of the scenes I was struggling with. I remember he wrote one scene about the rings on a tree and the passage of time that was really beautiful.

How did you learn the screenplay format? Did you see or read scripts growing up?

No, never. The truth is I don't read them now. I don't find it an enjoyable form to read, to be honest with you. I'm forced to read my own, and once in a while I will read someone else's, if I'm asked to do a rewrite or something; then you have no choice. But they're not literature, in most cases.

I was a reader for a while for [producer] Paul Monash, so I read scripts every day then.

The only script I remember that struck me and stuck with me was *Butch Cassidy and the Sundance Kid* (1969). I remember that was a script everybody felt was a piece of literature. Paul was the producer of *Butch Cassidy,* and I was a reader but also a development person for him for a certain period of time. I was involved—I don't say how involved—with *Butch Cassidy, Slaughterhouse Five* (1972), and *The Friends of Eddie Coyle* (1973).

There are two scripts that really changed the writing style of scripts. *Butch Cassidy* was one, because it had a sort of internal narrative like a novel, which almost poked fun at itself with parenthetical asides. The other one later on was *Lethal Weapon* (1987). Not the movie, the script. The *Lethal Weapon* script was famous—if there's any fame in this part of this world, the writing of screenplays—as pure action in a way that screenplays generally hadn't been written before. It was—and I don't mean this in a bad way—a sales presentation of what the movie was, with its own cool and hip language, very fast-paced, and short prose. You got a real sense of the movie.

I think that script was a by-product of movies of the '70s. A lot of scripts had that kind of feeling and were more stylistically oriented in the '70s, but they were less mainstream. *Lethal Weapon* was a mainstream movie and it popularized that style among scriptwriters.

The '60s had been more like the '50s in some respects, more inclined toward the old traditional studio system of script writing. You used to put in more format stuff and write scenes in terms of angles. You'd describe the camerawork and the succession of images more within the body of the scene. You'd write INTERIOR BEDROOM, CLOSE ANGLE, A CLOCK, MEDIUM ANGLE, A MAN ENTERS A ROOM. For whatever reasons, I don't know why, they used to feel writers should put in camera angles, so that's what I did too, starting out.

When did that drop off?

That didn't last much longer into the 1970s. I think most movies—not all—but a good bulk of the movies made in the '30s, '40s, and '50s were to some extent more like stage plays. They contained a lot more dialogue and weren't as visually oriented. That doesn't mean there weren't some great visual movies made then, but they weren't conceived in that way, per se. Some broke the mold, but there were, for lack of a better word, a lot of drawing-room-type pictures.

Besides the extra formatting and camera instructions, are there differences in your script style now, compared to those early scripts? Are you writing less dialogue, more description . . . anything like that? Has your style been evolving all along?

I don't feel like it has. I think I was always slightly novelistic in my style, with a lot of prose. I use descriptive sentences to give a sense of tone and a feeling of the piece. I don't think my style has changed that much. I write the same, long, dense scripts which people sometimes have criticized for their length. It's just the way I do it.

At the same time I was always praised by people who read my scripts, who said they could *see* the movie just from reading the script. They may not like the movie but, you know, they always got a sense of what it was. It's a little harder to do that with the more traditional screenplay form. In the more traditional screenplay form you have a little less prose. There's a shorthand and an architecture where you have to imagine things a bit more. Mine give more detail, not too much—I try to do a balance.

I don't feel like the way I write now is any different than the way I wrote then. Some of the techniques are a little different, and obviously I'm a little wiser and a better writer in some ways—at least I know how to do it better. But I have the same passions and there are certain ideas I wrote then that are still good ideas now.

• • •

When you were kicking around Hollywood in the late 1960s and early 1970s, meeting people, I wonder if you were having encounters with any of the old dinosaurs, the legendary Hollywood directors who were in the last stages of their lives and careers?

I met two people who were the most impressive to me. One was John Ford. When I made the documentary about the Poor People's March in 1968, we were editing it in a hole-in-the-wall room at the Samuel Goldwyn Studio, and I became friends with other people editing at that studio at the same time. I became quite close friends with Hal Ashby, who was also an editor, and with Barbara Ford, who was John Ford's daughter; she was an editor in one of rooms next to ours. In another room was Roman Polanski; I can't say he was a friend of mine, but he was there editing *Rosemary's Baby* (1968), so it was a great group.

Barbara Ford said, "Would you like to meet my father?" I said, "Are you joking?" I went home with her one night to the house. John—Mr. Ford—was in bed and had his famous eye patch on and all. It was, I want to say, 1969, or early 1970. I remember distinctly what the whole incident felt like. He was an old man, a gruff guy. I was wearing checkered bellbottoms, like you wore in those years. He said to me, "Step into the closeup. Are you wearing *checkered* pants?" *[laughs]*. I went there a few times just to talk to him about movies. We had great conversations.

The other director who I revered and met just by coincidence when I was working with Paul Monash was George Stevens—my office in that building was right above his. I had loved *Giant* (1956). It was a big influence on me. I like big American muscular movies with slightly melodramatic moments and great visuals, like Jet Rink, James Dean, standing under that oil well in *Giant*. I would run into George all the time and ask him all sorts of questions about movies. George was at that time preparing *The Only Game in Town* (1970), which I love; it was written by Frank Gilroy. George was a magnificent director, and as nice a man as I ever met.

How did The Nickel Ride *evolve?*

That was an original idea of mine. It was originally called "50–50." It was supposed to be about a man who is turning fifty, a film noir with intimations of mortality. As a matter of fact, Quentin Tarantino has said it is one of the better American film noir movies.

You were a fan of film noir.

Very much so. Anyway I just decided I wanted to write it, and then the script made its way through an agent and a couple of people to Robert Mulligan, the director.

It originally had gone to George C. Scott, who was interested in playing the lead. He was at the same agency as Robert Mulligan, the William Morris Agency, and I think George C. Scott may have given Bob the script. Anyway it didn't work out with George C. Scott—he got sick, or something happened—I don't think it was a creative problem. I wish he had done it. But he went off to be in something else, and Bob stayed with the script and made the movie.

It was a big break for me because I only had had that one other movie made, which was a very small, very forgettable, little love story. Now I was working with an important director. And I got a more important agent, because I did what most people do—I took advantage of the fact that I could jump to the William Morris Agency, a bigger, more powerful agency.

What did Robert Mulligan do to make your script better or worse?

Oh, he made it better. We collaborated very closely. The only thing that might have made the movie—I don't know about better—certainly different, was that George C. Scott was supposed to play the lead, and I think it would have been amazing with him in the part. Scott left, and then Bob cast it differently. The guy who ended up playing the character really was younger than the part called for: the young actor Jason Miller, who was in *The Exorcist* (1973), and who was also a playwright; he won the Pulitzer for *That Championship Season.* A good man.

I ended up doing a couple of scripts for Bob. That's the only one that got made.

I know you got very busy after Nickel Ride *but your official credits are sparse for most of the rest of the 1970s. I gather you spent much of that decade as a ghostwriter or fix-it writer on numerous films, without credit. Why is that?*

That's a good question. It just fell that way. One reason is that I never really particularly fought for credit on films. I can give you examples of six, seven movies that people probably don't even know I had anything to do with. You'd have to go project by project. Each one has its own story.

For example, I rewrote *The Drowning Pool.* That's because I was friends with Stuart Rosenberg. I came in after somebody else had written the first script, so I felt that that film was theirs and not mine. I didn't think I had done enough to merit credit. Nowadays, I don't know if I would have gotten credit for my work, or not. Probably yes. I did some other work for Stuart over the years, on *The Pope of Greenwich Village* and other films. When you have relationships with certain directors, you're not always doing full-out work where you deserve credit. But I didn't think of myself as a script doctor, or fix-it writer. I find that sort of insulting.

Another example: *The Onion Field,* on which I'm uncredited. I'm sure I would have won credit if I had fought for it in that case. I was quite friendly with Michael Douglas and I was offered to do *One Flew Over the Cuckoo's*

Nest (1975), and simultaneously I was offered to do *The Onion Field.* My agent in his wisdom—I'm not saying he was wrong, because at that point it looked like *Cuckoo's Nest* might not even get made—advised me to do *Onion Field.* So I decided to do *Onion Field,* which is something I regretted for a long time. After I did my version of *Onion Field,* they were unable to go forward for various reasons—there was a problem with the producers and the director—then Joe Wambaugh came back in and he, with the producers, was able to move it to another director and writer. At that point, I don't know why, I didn't fight for credit.

I never did a draft of *Cuckoo's Nest,* but I did a couple of scenes for the producers and I met with Milos Forman. They asked me back a couple of times, but not enough where I would deserve credit. So I guess you would call that ghostwriting, but it wasn't really. They ended up getting Bo Goldman, who is a great writer. A couple little ideas of mine remained in the film.

There were a few of those situations. There was another movie I did called *Wolfen,* where I didn't fight for credit, and I could almost guarantee I would have gotten credit on *Wolfen.*

I mean half of it was my own culpability of coming in on other people's work, or sometimes people coming in on my work. The other half was I just didn't have any big feeling about sharing in the credits. I don't know why, but at that point in time I didn't give a shit. I don't remember people actually fighting over credits then, either. Maybe the bonuses weren't the same. Credits have come to mean more now in certain respects. And I'm not saying they don't mean anything to me, but I don't have the same feeling about credits as some people do.

Also, I was not an "A" writer during that period of time. There was a group of bigger-name writers and old-timers, and then you had whatever my group was. We weren't necessarily "B" writers but we weren't the people getting movies made. The "A" group included some people who became well known and had a great body of work—people like Robert Towne—and they didn't put their names on rewrites either. You felt that unless you were really proud of something, what was the point of putting your name on it? That doesn't mean it wasn't a good movie, as I've said; it had to do with pride of authorship, at least for me. I can tell you, Bob Towne did tons of rewriting without taking credit. They were just not films that he felt were his.

They made movies differently then. Very independent during that era. A little less scripted. A little more improvisational. In some respects they were not doing the sort of movies I'd be more apt to write. I was more interested in structured, traditionally dramatic movies.

Was it frustrating not to be credited? Did it bother you at all at the time?

I don't think I really cared, oddly. Isn't that odd? None of those movies I felt were mine. *Onion Field,* for example, I thought was a good movie, not a great movie. I like my version of *Onion Field* better than the movie they made. And I had pride of authorship for the parts I'd written.

Was it partly that there was more production and steady work? So steady work was good work.

I don't know. I'm being honest with you. The reason was, I think, I was young, I was getting stoned, I was enjoying working, I was lucky to get regular work, and I was always busy. I got to choose what I did. My strong suit was, I think, my salary was a little lower than other people so I think they got a good bargain for their money. But they paid me well, and I had a good life. It was a good time to be a screenwriter. And maybe because nothing resulted entirely from a script of mine, I didn't really feel that huge a pride of authorship in any of the films.

. . .

Your circumstances begin to change, certainly the credits begin to line up differently, starting in the late 1970s, with The Concorde . . . Airport '79, Memories of Me, Suspect, *and* Mr. Jones. *How did it happen that you ended up collaborating with Billy Crystal on* Memories of Me?

When I was at Universal—doing the *Airport* movie actually—I was on the same hall as the management firm called Rollins and Joffe, who handled all sorts of huge comedians, particularly Woody Allen and a director named Steve Gordon, who made *Arthur* (1981). We were all friends, and it was wild times. Stu Smiley, a young manager for Charlie Joffe, thought Billy and I would like each other, and he introduced us and we did like each other. I had this idea for a script based on a relative of mine, a great uncle who was a professional extra. I told Billy about this guy and my idea, and he thought it was attractive, and together we came up with the story. Billy would come over after working on *Soap* [the 1977–81 TV series] and we would sit and write at night.

How was it writing with Billy Crystal? Kind of like a fast tennis game?

It was easy. It was fun! The movie didn't work out too good *[laughs]*. I think it just wasn't as well realized as maybe it could have been.

Billy plays a very sour character. His father is the more likable character, even though the audience is supposed to be wary of the father.

Yeah, I know. I don't want to take Henry Winkler to task, but he's not a director. I think it could have been a moving movie.

Suspect *was your first solo credit since* Nickel Ride. *How did that come about?*

The industry was changing slightly. And I was friendly with Jeff Sagansky, who was president of TriStar, so I had a good deal with that studio. TriStar, at that time, seemed to like whatever I wrote, so nobody touched my scripts. That was important for the credits.

I had been working with a producer who wanted to make a film out of a book by a woman named Linda Wolfe, who wrote very good crime books, all true stories. One was an extremely complicated case about a guy who was a man, who became a woman, and then she as a he, or he as a she, killed the lover of his ex-wife—a real crazy gender-confused case. I loved it as a case. The system was tested by the case, and the whole story was anarchistic. I never wrote any script, but the producer kept trying to get the project off the ground. We never had any luck.

When my involvement fell by the wayside I still was interested in the whole notion of the courtroom being "suspect"—in quotes—rather than "a suspect," which ended up becoming the title of the eventual movie. I didn't have anything else to do, so I thought I would try to write an original in which the system was tested by a strange murder case. I like the man who directed it, a nice man who made some good movies, Peter Yates—but I don't think he ever quite got this one down on film.

I rather enjoyed the movie.

The ending is cheeseball, though.

There's something about Cher playing the lead that doesn't add up.

It's the wrong part for her but there are a lot of good actors in the film. It's the first American part for Liam Neeson. Joe Mantegna is in it. John Mahoney plays the villain. Peter Yates is quite talented, but if I had to do it over again I'd change the ending.

Oddly, the movie did fairly well, but we were hurt by the fact that it came out at the same time as *Fatal Attraction* (1987). It's a decent, solid, maybe clunky melodrama.

How did Mr. Jones *evolve?*

After *Suspect,* which as I said did pretty well, TriStar said to me, "What do you want to write next?" I said I'd like to do a Hitchcock-type medical thriller like *Spellbound.* I did some research about mental illness and manic depression, and I realized I didn't want to do this subject as a melodrama. I wanted to do it as a serious dramatic movie. That's what I set out to do, writing the script. Richard Gere got involved, Ray Stark got involved, and then this certain director came on who I didn't like at all—and he and I had big fights.

My wife [Debra Greenfield] was actually the producer of *Mr. Jones.* There's a great story attached to it. We were sitting in our den one day and the phone rang and she answered it. "Blah, blah, blah." She hung up and said, "You're fired." "What are you talking about?" Anyway the director didn't want me to work on the film anymore. He ended up getting fired himself, so fuck him.

Then they brought Mike Figgis on as the director and the situation kind of spiraled. It happens. My script was rewritten by Michael Cristofer.

So you and the first director stayed fired, but your wife stayed producer?

Well, I actually came back to do some rewriting and became friends with somebody else who did some rewriting on it—Barbara Benedek, who's a wonderful writer. But the movie was neither fish nor fowl. Some of it was very good, and some of it was silly. I think Michael Cristofer did a good job, but, to me, the movie fell way short. Too many hands got in the middle.

The original script was pretty great, I have to say. There was a lovely moment in the original script that they never used which I actually put in another movie.

Is it a secret?

It's a total subtlety in *The Good Shepherd.*

In *Mr. Jones,* he at one point tells his psychiatrist about a dream he has supposedly had about a room with a curtain that has a certain fabric on it, et cetera, et cetera. She starts thinking this may not be a dream, it might be something that was part of his life experience. She goes to Berkeley, where he had gone to school, and finds out where he lived then. She walks along the street, looks up, sees this curtain. She goes upstairs and the room is completely as it was, twenty years earlier. The apartment manager tells her someone pays the rent every month. It's where Mr. Jones first became sick. I thought it was a quite chilling, quite lovely moment.

In *The Good Shepherd* there's a scene where they point out a certain clue, curtains that are made with baobab-tree patterns, and, later, the Matt Damon character is walking along a street, he looks up and he sees the curtains with the baobab pattern. So it's the same image.

. . .

*When did you first hear those two auspicious words—*Forrest Gump*?*

It was just a piece of work that came to me. Wendy Finerman, who was the producer of the project, gave me the book, and she simultaneously gave it to Tom Hanks, who was a longtime friend of mine. Wendy, Tom, and I had all been working on *The Postman,* I'm afraid to say, lo, those many years ago. Tom was involved with *The Postman* and was possibly going to star in the film, which was written as a satire before becoming an earnest mess of a movie nine years later, when I was no longer involved with it.

Anyway, Wendy gave us this book she had been developing at Warner Brothers. She had had a couple of scripts written, which I never read. I read the book, and I thought there was a good spirit to it, if a little farcical for my taste.

Did the project come to you in part because it wasn't high profile and you weren't a high-profile screenwriter at that time?

Yes, I think that's true, but I liked the fact that a bunch of people had failed trying to do it. I thought it was a challenge and I knew I could do whatever I wanted to do with it because it wasn't a real viable project.

So you and Tom read the book at the same time.

Yes, simultaneously. I said to Tom, "I think I have a way to do this . . ." He said, "Really?" I said, "Would you be willing to try this if I can write it?" He said, "Yeah, I'm in." So he was in before I wrote anything, and then he continued to be an inspiration.

Rather than Warner Brothers stepping forward, they decided to put it in turnaround and Wendy took it to Paramount, where Brandon Tartikoff, rest his soul, was the new president of the studio. Tom Hanks and I went in and pitched it together. It was a big advantage having Tom there, because he could act out certain things that I told him I was planning to do.

Did that first pitch have all that scope of the eventual movie?

I think it did. I had thought it out. There had been another director who was briefly on board whom I had spoken to about it—Barry Sonnenfeld. I gave him some ideas and that opened up my thinking. Barry was potentially involved with *The Postman* and for a time he was potentially involved with *Forrest Gump,* which didn't work out in either case.

Oddly, on the spot during the pitch I came up with this idea of the feather—an old man sitting on a bench and a feather landing there, a symbol of fate. The feather was reminiscent to me of the timeless quality of the opening of *The World According to Garp* (1982), the movie—the baby bouncing—and also the Coen brothers with the hat rolling in *Miller's Crossing* (1990). I love that idea of the arbitrary nature of fate. The book had *Forrest Gump* sitting on a bus bench at the beginning and I went further with that, where he would be sitting on the bench throughout the film and telling everybody who comes along his story, allowing us to go back and forth in time.

The bus-bench scene in the book has the piece-of-candy line, only it's a throwaway and not the credo it becomes in the film.

The line in the book is, "Life is no box of chocolates." Later, when discussing the script to Bob Zemeckis, I said, "Life is like a box of chocolates," and he said to me, "What are you talking about?" I said, "You never know what you are going to get." That's how the line was born.

My feeling, from the outside looking in, is that if you and Tom went into a pitch meeting with an important studio official, that it would be a relatively easy sell.

Even though Tom was a star, he certainly wasn't a star like he is now, or became. He hadn't done *Sleepless in Seattle* (1993) or *Philadelphia* (1993) yet. He had had a bit of a lull in his career. At that point, he couldn't just pick out what he wanted to do. They could have said no and we would have understood that. But Brandon felt kindly toward the project and said let's develop it.

How much did you improvise during the pitch?

They were familiar with the book. They had the coverage. I walked in and said I have an approach to this that I think could be very funny, very touching, that involves this man of a low IQ who would like to be normal, who is sitting on a bench relating his life story, which is slightly unbelievable but happens to be true—sort of like the unbelievable things that have happened in all our own lifetimes—with the real incidents sometimes being more unbelievable than anything I could make up. And I talked about our generation growing older, looking back on past times and what those times meant to us, and what was important to people, et cetera, et cetera.

Some improvisation, and some things I had thought about. Like I said, the feather idea dawned on me, although I *had* thought about it; but when I was sitting there I decided I may as well give it a whirl. I gave some examples of the things I wanted to do. Tom acted out a few bits. He had some version of that *Forrest Gump* accent, and some things he did were very funny.

Were you already talking about the soundtrack as the music of the '60s?

Oh yeah, completely. I'd already thought that out too. But you don't give away too much when you do these pitches. You give a general sense of the movie. The main inspiration was Forrest Gump on a park bench and the feather and the story shifting back and forth in time. Brandon said yes, and then it was up to me to execute.

It's a beautifully written novel—and it really surprised me reading it, how different it is from the movie. Is there a way you can encapsulate your contribution to turning the book into the film?

I think that the film doesn't exist without me, if you want me to be totally arrogant.

[Laughs.] *Yes, I do.*

I don't agree with you about the book. I don't think it's so beautifully written. I was troubled by the book because of the farcical nature of it, because in the novel Forrest weighed three hundred pounds, he goes to the moon with a monkey, and other crazy episodes. I guess you could find it funny. It wasn't my sense of humor. But there was also this sadness about the book, and it reminded me of the [John Kennedy] Toole book, *A Confederacy of Dunces* (1980). Both Southern books with an abiding sadness about the main character. And the character grew on me, I don't know why, I had no relationship to this character particularly, in my life.

Do you have to find some personal way into the script you're writing?

I absolutely do. It has to be something I want to talk about, something I feel I'm able to say. Yes, completely. Otherwise I feel alien to the material and I just couldn't write it.

One of the things that must have helped you was the historical context of Gump. *The character in the book does live through the '60s and gets his picture taken with famous people, but you have him interact more with the '60s, rather than, in the book, going to the moon and later becoming marooned on a Pacific island. You brought the '60s into his story in a much broader and, it seems to me, more personal way. I find it a serious movie about the '60s.*

It is, of a certain kind. Zemeckis has a sense of humor that is slightly cynical, and he likes to poke people in the eye of all political flavors. So it was a look at some of the excesses of the '60s, or at least our narcissism in certain areas, and on the other hand it was about the core values of the '60s which I think were good, and about all sorts of people in that era.

Anyway the book was fun but it didn't sell many copies and was generally forgotten. And so whatever unique ideas I came up with are reflected in the movie.

Was the producer looking for a faithful rendition of the book?

No, she didn't have any specific ideas like that. She had found this quirky, weird book and trusted me do something with it.

Was there any question of involving the novelist Winston Groom, or talking to him at all?

He wanted to be involved, but I was the one who was stubborn about that. The property had not worked in many incarnations, including the book. I mean, it didn't sell well. I felt I had been asked to write a movie and that is what I know about. Down the road he was very happy.

How long did it take you once you went to the typewriter?

Usually scripts take me about a year, so basically, about a year.

A year from the first draft to the final draft.

A year for the draft. A year from when I first set pen to paper, or typewriter to paper, for the first draft.

No one was supervising you during that year of writing?

That's the way I work anyway. I go off and work. I tell people generally what I'm going to write and I get some feedback, but I don't often sit and listen to people as I'm writing.

The three main characters from the book remain basically the same in the film. But you jettisoned so much of the novel's storyline, replacing it with your own narrative. Did you encounter much resistance to that?

Quite honestly, nobody ever knew. Until I turned the script in I don't know how anyone could have known. I might have said to the producer, "I'm going off in my own direction here," but she said good luck.

When you sit down to write, do you have it blocked out structurally in some form on paper?

Not really. That one was a little complicated because I had to go back and forth in time. I always know the beginning and the ending of a script, and I know I started out with Forrest Gump as a young boy and the braces he had to wear. The story started to fill itself in by the chronology of events in his life. I don't write from an outline too much. It grows by its own volition. I might outline two or three scenes ahead in my head, or write them down: one, two, three.

You don't have any note cards, or outline? What is your theory, that if you can't remember something it isn't worth remembering?

It's mostly in my head. I write little things down on scraps of paper—just a line of dialogue, or a description. But I usually remember what I'm planning to write.

I have a tremendous memory, especially my visual memory. I can remember how things looked forty years ago, right down to the exact details—what was on the desk, what people were wearing, how the weather was. Like a photograph. I'm a little savantey that way.

Do you have any tricks for writing dialogue? Do you speak it out?

I do speak it out in some corny voice of my own, trying to say each person's part. I sort of say it halfway aloud, almost unconsciously, since if I were to think about it I'd be embarrassing myself.

Were you putting specific music and songs in the script?

Yes and no. I made references not to specific songs but to where we could utilize music from different periods.

The film has one of the all-time pop music scores.

That was Bob Zemeckis as much as anyone; Bob, along with a guy named Joel Sill, picked out the music and they had a whole conception of doing top-twenty hits from those years.

Instead of going to outer space Forrest jogs cross-country. Where did the idea of Forrest running come from?

Running, jogging, marathons were becoming part of the culture, and I lived in San Diego where it was already part of the culture. I understood people doing it for health reasons, but running was also a great metaphor. People running, but where are they running to? I had a slightly cynical outlook about running, because, although I know it's good for your health, on the other hand some people in the yuppie generation were running for no particular reasons—just to run. I felt it would be a plausible activity for a guy who has no other skills. So it was meant to be slightly humorous but also as a way for him to do something cathartic. At the same time running takes him—and the audience—across the country so they can witness various episodes.

When the film came out, it was criticized by some people for what they saw as its satirical attitude toward the Movement of the 1960s. Not that I agree with that criticism.

Well, I think those people have no sense of humor, number one; they take themselves too seriously. Number two, as I said, Bob Zemeckis is an equal opportunity eye poker. His politics were a little more right wing than mine. I can't say what his politics are particularly, but I think he takes a more jaundiced view. He wasn't as enamored of the '60s as I might have been.

Did he do any writing at all? Because he of course started out as a writer and had his own reputation for scripts like Used Cars *(1980) and the* Back to the Future *series.*

No. We were collegial. It was a collaboration. After Bob got involved we sat and talked for a while and I had to rewrite the draft. The original script had all sorts of cartoonish ideas in it that were imaginative but probably overkill. I had Forrest seeing images associated with certain people, for example. Lieutenant Dan always had a black cloud over his head—literally—that lifted when he found God. Jenny, she always had angel wings. They were interesting conceits, but Bob felt—and he turned out to be right—we should take them out. He cut out the excesses where I went overboard. There were some excesses, I've got to admit.

Bob worked the way a director should, asking, "Why is this scene like this?" We'd discuss scenes, and I'd go rewrite them. But it's a good shorthand when the director is also a writer, because you don't have to prove yourself on certain questions. He understands the language.

How long did that process of working with Zemeckis and the rewriting take?

Another three to four months, maybe.

Did Tom get more involved at that point?

Definitely, although he wasn't involved per se until Bob and I had gotten the script to where Bob was happy with it. Then we went to Tom, and Tom would say, "Why am I doing this? Why am I saying this?" We then sat at a table with the other actors, same thing, and I would fix those concerns. They might say, "I could probably say this better this way," or "I could do this with a look," or "I'm uncomfortable with saying this, it's too on-the-nose for me." Actors always ask good questions, and you'd better figure out how to answer their questions. Things would change out of those discussions. It's a process, it always is.

Does the process stop when the filming starts?

That depends on the director. Bob, on *Forrest Gump*, was very specific, very organized, a very bottom-line kind of guy, in a good way. He told me—I don't remember the exact dates—but that I'd be doing writing until August whatever and then they'd start shooting in late August. By then we'd gone through a number of versions of the script. We'd gone through everybody giving their input—the actors—and what needed to be changed depending on locations and budgetary needs and everything else. They had had read-throughs and rehearsals, and I was there, and changes came out of those stages too. Two to three weeks before we started shooting, I was done. There were maybe two or three little tiny things I had to do during shooting.

With other directors it's different. With some people I've been involved all the way through.

So you're done with the writing, and they go ahead with the filming—and gradually the music and special effects are added. What is the point at which you see the film that has been made from your script?

Again, it depends on the director. With Bob I wasn't invited to the editing at all. That was his purview. But I had seen a lot because we had to do narration, and so he ran the movie for me alone, once I think, and then once with Tom, as he was putting it together, so we could get a sense of what we might have to change or add to the narration. Then Tom started doing looping, and I was there every day helping with the narration, so on the spot we would rewrite bits or I would go home and fix things for the next day. I got to see a lot of the movie that way.

Then we started previewing it. I went to all the previews and we'd discuss the audience reactions.

When did you begin to get the sense that it was going to be such a big movie? Was the idea growing on your that you had something unusual on your hands?

Yes, especially after the first screening, because it tested so well. The second one tested higher, and the third one even higher. Then we were on an airplane coming back from San Jose and a screening at a huge theater that Bob always uses, and one of the execs who knows how to read all these cards said, "Well, your scores have just gone to *Indiana Jones* territory." When you watched the movie with an audience you got the sense that it was, for lack of a better word, magical.

You've had a lot of success, but Gump *has had the biggest box-office returns. In some way it touched many more people than any of your other movies.*

Certainly *Gump* was the most successful. No question about it: look, it's part of the lexicon. It's an iconic movie. People mention it all the time. Every day. That's lovely.

Was Gump *the script of yours most perfectly filmed?*

No, there have been a number. I think *The Insider* is about as close as you can get to something I'd written. *The Good Shepherd* is. *The Curious Case of Benjamin Button,* from what I've seen, definitely is.

Forrest Gump I'd find less fault with, for whatever reasons. It's not because of the success of the movie. I think Bob captured the ironic quality of it, almost to a T. He did a great job of editing the script and maintaining the tone of the piece. I don't think it's the greatest movie ever made, no. Is it a wonderful piece of work? Yes.

. . .

How did your life change after Forrest Gump? *Did your price go way up and the offers come flooding in?*

Obviously I was sought after.

Did it change the way you wrote?

No, I don't think so.

Did it make you nervous, raising the stakes on your next script?

Briefly you think you're king of the world, but that's ridiculous. Shortly after the Oscars—this is amusing—I went to work for Robert Redford and he basically said to me, "What have you done for *me* lately?" So you start from square one in that sense. Each assignment, each new script, is a challenge, and people expect you to hit the ball out of the ballpark.

Curiously, The Postman *was your next major credit. I have to admit I don't think it turned out so terrible.*

Well, who can account for bad taste *[laughs]*? I had literally written it nine years earlier, and it was supposed to be a satirical look at the postapocalypse. Tom Hanks was going to be the star. It was even going to open up with the Lou Reed song, "And the colored girls go boop-de-boop-de-boop . . ." That was the whole tone of the script. Kevin Costner made an utterly earnest movie that didn't reflect what I wanted. Even if it had been successful, it wasn't what I wanted.

The only reason I have credit on *The Postman*—aside from maybe I deserve it, even though they changed the whole plot and tone—is that it was rewritten by a man named Brian Helgeland, who went on to win an Oscar for *L.A. Confidential* (1997) and who is a friend of mine. He was very generous and said he would share credit with me, or he could have solo credit, or I could have solo credit. I was conflicted, and we left it the way it was: a shared credit. The movie's not something I'm very proud of.

Did Redford and The Horse Whisperer *come along because of* Forrest Gump *or irrespective of* Forrest Gump?

There was a producer who worked for Bob named Rachel Pfeffer, and she was a fan of my scripts. So it wasn't strictly *Forrest Gump,* even though I was very hirable.

The impression I get of Redford is that he nurtures a lot of properties, ponders and weighs them, and moves very slowly toward realizing a film, especially when he is directing.

He's very cautious about what he does. He takes a long time between projects. He's a very thoughtful guy, very methodical, intelligent about his decisions. It was a complicated relationship for me. I like him personally. The work relationship had some great aspects, and some aspects I didn't like as much, but that's always true about personalities you work with.

I would think it was different for you, coming so soon after Forrest Gump, *in that when Redford adapts a book into a film generally he's trying to be very faithful to the book.*

To some extent, except for there were various parts of that story where we weren't sure what to do and some parts from the book that wouldn't work as well translated into a movie. The truth is, after quite a long period of time, I ran out of gas on that project. Bob probably did the right thing by bringing in another writer, because I don't think I was serving his needs at that point.

There are ways in which the film seems in search of a proper ending.

The book didn't really have a very satisfying ending. I don't like to judge the film. It became what it became and Bob was happy with it, I assume, and I was glad I was able to make a contribution. I'm not trying to deflect blame here but that's the way the game is played. I saw the piece one way, the way I wrote it, and he wanted a vision more to his taste.

But the film is still your vision to a great extent, right?

Oh yes, well past fifty percent. But it's the book's also, and these films become a blend of many influences. I'm proud of much original writing that's still in the movie. The scene where the character Bob plays waits for the horse to come back, for example, is mine. I'm not tooting my own horn but I think it was a lovely scene and captured the essence of the piece. And many other ideas in the film are mine. But many parts came from the book or from Richard LaGravenese, who is a good writer. It's unhappy, obviously, when you don't finish a project because you want to finish it for your own sake, professionally, and for all sorts of reasons.

What is your background with Michael Mann?

Michael and I go back years. He had read a version of *The Good Shepherd,* which I first wrote after *Forrest Gump,* and he was impressed by it. We met to talk about that script. Michael was thinking of directing *The Good Shepherd,* but that didn't work out and we kept in communication. We respected each other's creativity, I guess you'd say, and I like Michael personally very much. Then *The Insider* came along.

Michael had been friends and gone to school with Lowell Bergman, the journalist, who, along with me and Michael, simultaneously had a deal at the Walt Disney Studio. Michael had bought the magazine article about Lowell and *60 Minutes* that Marie Brenner had written in *Vanity Fair,* and he brought it to me. I read it and said, "I'm not sure I'm the right guy for this. It's a little out of my ken, this kind of docudrama writing." But Michael persisted. Michael's persistent.

Why did you think it was out of your ken?

It wasn't like anything I had done. I wasn't sure I could do it. Not that I was disinterested, it was just different for me and I didn't feel like it was something I could do naturally. But Michael said give it a whirl and he won the day. I wrote a bunch of pages, he loved them, and that gave me confidence to go ahead. Then he came on with me and we wrote together.

There can't have been that much drama—at least cinematic drama—in the original magazine piece.

There was drama of a kind. It was an unlikely subject for a movie because it's not, on face value, something that would seem compelling.

It's probably the least likely subject for any Hollywood film for years.

I must say for degree of difficulty—they're all difficult—that was probably the hardest one. I was very satisfied that we were able to make it work.

I would have thought as you went around Hollywood and told people what film you were writing people would have said, "Are you kidding?"

Basically they did, except for Joe Roth, who was running Disney at the time, and who had great faith in Michael. The creative work is attributable to both of us, but the film is attributable to Michael. He had a dog-with-a-bone attitude about making that film, and a strong point of view. That movie got made because of him, not anything else.

Was it absolutely vital to have a star to give it some lift at the box office?

Russell Crowe was known as a good actor but he didn't really carry any weight. Al Pacino is certainly a star and it was valuable to have him. Michael probably would have gotten it done anyway but with lesser money, and Al was right for the role—plus he was wonderful.

At the end of The Insider *there is a crawl that says the film is blended fact and fiction. What kind of responsibility—especially with Michael Mann being friends with Lowell Bergman—do you have to the reality? I think the film is tough on everybody but in the end, of course, Lowell Bergman comes off as quite heroic. What is your responsibility to the facts?*

That's always the great conundrum: drama and art versus reality. I feel my first job is to be a dramatist. I'm not trying to make a documentary. I want to be as accurate as possible to what happened in reality, and if I can't be, then at least I want to give a sense of what happened and be thematically true to what happened. You have a great moral responsibility to be accurate and honest. You can't fly in the face of the truth. But it's a real tightrope walk as to when you are taking too many liberties.

Is that one reason why the job was so daunting? That you had this extra layer of responsibility, other than relying on your imagination?

Yes and no. As an artist you can take certain liberties, while at the same time there's a definite responsibility to stay within the confines of the truth as best you can. But there are various versions of truth. Everybody has a different point of view. If you are writing the characters of Lowell Bergman and Mike Wallace, both have different points of view about what happened in the story we were telling. Not that I come in to settle that argument, because at any moment I might be taking one point of view over the other, or trying to strike a balance. I'm less interested in trying to solve the issues than I am in treating a character and his beliefs fairly.

If I'm writing "Mike Wallace," I try to separate myself from the real Mike Wallace. I tell myself I'm writing an eighty-year-old (or whatever his age was), world-renowned (and certainly justifiably so) journalist. I say to myself, "What do I imagine are his emotions, his fears?" So I start creating a character that isn't really him. Hopefully the character is representative of some things Mike Wallace happens to be, but there will be other things about the character the real Mike Wallace may resent. They become characters. They're not those people, per se. It's a tightrope walk.

Even Mike Wallace himself, when he sits in front of the camera and asks questions, he's "Mike Wallace, the interviewer." He's not "Mike Wallace, the solo person."

That sense of a divided self comes across in the movie as well. Did you interact with Mike Wallace while writing the film, that is, study him or follow him at close quarters?

Only telephone calls. He would call and yell at me. I would take whatever he said and put it into the movie.

How would he know to yell at you?

He had actually got a copy of the script at one point.

How about Lowell Bergman? Did you interact with him, study him?

We're good friends. We became good friends. We are still very good friends. Actually, if I had to do it again, I would show Lowell as having more weaknesses. At that point in time I didn't really know him as well as I know him now. If there's a criticism of the film, it may be that I wasn't balanced enough in his portrait, and I should have been. I think that's a fair criticism.

How much research do you typically do? I suppose you had to do some research on Forrest Gump *even, considering that the film touched on so much history and so many factual events.*

Forrest Gump didn't really require much research. I lived through all those things, so that didn't require much at all. In general I research as I go. There's a benefit to research and there's a detraction. There's a balance you have to strike.

So if you run into a scene with a hole or a gap, that is when you might stop and do a little research?

Not so much if you run into a factual problem, but you have to get some details right in order to know how people would react in a certain way because of the reality of a situation. My process is I start with a theme, normally, and then I'm interested in how the characters and the story will relate to that theme. The facts have to be balanced with the theme.

How about in the case of Ali?

Ali required a lot of research, even though I knew a lot about Ali because I used to box when I was younger.

You were a boxer?

I boxed in college and I boxed in Golden Gloves when I was a kid growing up in Brooklyn.

The burden wasn't history in that case; for that movie it was the burden of the sheer personality of the real human being, and how people relate to him. I think Will Smith did a great, great job, but he could never be Ali. There's a magnetism about the real Ali which you can't quite capture, so the movie tried to talk about other things: What was the responsibility this guy had and what it did to him as a man; what that responsibility did to his personal life; and what kind of burden it is to carry the world around on your shoulders.

Was that the theme in your head before you started on Ali?

That one was handed to me, Thematically, that was not so much my idea, as it was a combination of Michael Mann and I. We both agreed this was a story we wanted to tell. The theme was a hard one to articulate, but basically within the movie we wanted to explore the question: what does it mean to be Muhammad Ali? As with most of Michael's movies, it was a very interior profile of someone. In Michael's movies, normally, you're looking at someone from inside out—psychologically, emotionally, and everything else. While in my other movies, it's the other way around, you're sometimes looking in. Most movies, actually, look in rather than look out.

Michael had decided in a brief moment to do *Ali.* He called me and said, "We've got to move, I need a script in six or eight weeks," which is unheard-of for me—since it usually takes me a year. We both started writing. There had been a script that existed, but it was not the story we wanted to tell. It was a decent script, it just wasn't how we saw the film. So I was given a different kind of instructions. It wasn't like, "Let's sit and bullshit and talk about Muhammad Ali and how we want to tell a story"—setting a leisurely pace and taking a year to do all the research you might want to do. It was instead really heavy lifting and a lot of hard labor.

And you had to do it in six or eight weeks?

Yeah, in six or eight weeks.

Were you writing together in the same room?

No. On *The Insider* it was a little different. I wrote a version of the script and then I sat down and went over it scene by scene with Michael. Then we'd flip and switch scenes. Michael would play with some scenes and I'd rewrite others. It became more of a collaboration.

Ali was collaborative from the beginning. I wrote the first two acts and he wrote the third, and then we swapped because we were in a big hurry. And that is the draft we had when we started filming, and then we would work on polishing scenes every day.

Is that unusual for you?

Yes, very unusual.

Because generally you write alone.

I still did, even with Michael. We didn't spend time writing together. I would send him pages, he would give me his reaction.

He's a formidable screenwriter in his own right.

A very good writer. We write differently. I have different strengths than him. We were able, at least on those two movies, to work well together. And there's another one we're trying to get made, which I wrote for him after *Ali*, called "Commanche," a western, which I think is potentially spectacular. Michael has put his two cents in, and now we're coming to some conclusions about it. It keeps moving a little closer to fruition.

Anyway, as I've said, *Ali* was problematic because so much was already known about Ali, he's such a public persona. The challenge was to tell a story that hadn't been told before and also to try and find a theme that would reflect our feelings about Ali's life, his relationship with different people, and his relationship to the world. It was a massive undertaking.

Did Ali himself sign off on it? Were you interacting with him constantly?

Yes, yes. He was on the set much of the time, and so were the people around him. He has marvelous people who look out for him, and he can look out for himself to a certain extent. We were very attuned to the myth and the real man, and we tried to portray both. We also tried to dramatize various key events and important relationships he had with well-known people like Malcolm X. It was daunting on the one hand, and on the other it was a labor of love.

I still feel, personally, that we didn't quite get the third act right, which is not Michael's fault or mine. Something didn't quite mesh. I wish we would have had more time. We succeeded to a great degree and not entirely. But I'm not sure we ever could have succeeded entirely. I'm not sure you could ever capture the personality of Muhammad Ali. He's bigger than all of us.

. . .

What brought Spielberg to you on Munich*?*

I started to get offered a lot of serious dramatic projects after *The Insider* and *Ali*. But I'd known Steven for years and years. We've always been respectful of one another. We had a couple of near-misses on projects. *Forrest Gump*, oddly, he was interested in, and *The Curious Case of Benjamin Button*, too; he read *The Good Shepherd* and we had a long talk about that script at one point, though I don't think he was interested in directing it. He was familiar with my work.

I had been working with Kathleen Kennedy on *Benjamin Button*, and she was also one of the producers on *Munich*. They wanted a rewrite on a draft, which was supposed to take a month or six weeks of work. It turned into a year of my life.

Who were you rewriting?

David and Janet Peoples; David wrote *Unforgiven* (1992). They had done a very full, very long first draft and, I don't know why, they didn't continue and I was brought on to work closely with Steven.

I would think the research-historical burden of working on Munich *would be the toughest of all.*

Steven was the glue on that movie, no question about it. It was all about whatever Steven wanted. We had interesting intellectual or creative fights about it—in good ways.

Was Steven doing actual writing too?

He writes with his directorial style. It's all writing, quite honestly. Screenwriters can give a blueprint or provide architecture, and certainly they give the dramatis personae, but it's still a blueprint. When you're directing you're writing; when you're acting you're writing; editing is certainly writing. It's all writing. Hopefully it's in service of what you've written to begin with.

Emotionally the film was hard, because I had mixed emotions about it. And it was hard because we were trying to combine an intelligent, thoughtful, emotional dramatic movie with a very high bar of integrity. We were trying to create the kinds of scenes you need to have in movies—suspense, action sequences, those kinds of scenes—while maintaining a high integrity and staying as close as possible to the truth, or at least as we knew the truth to be.

When you say mixed emotions, do you mean . . .

It has to do with my own feelings about Israel. Some days I'd feel as if the Israelis were not behaving the way I hoped they would, and other days, obviously, the Palestinians would blow up children on a school bus and I would just say, "Fuck 'em. Kill every one of 'em."

Those conflicted feelings come across in the trajectory of the main character, and they are echoed in audiences' reactions to the movie.

I know, I know. And that's how Steven felt about the subject too. That's why the story and the whole moral imperative of the movie is really interesting and very important. The question being, as normal men, when are we doing the right or wrong thing, and how far should we go? When does certain behavior become immoral? There are obviously lots of issues involved in the film.

There again I went to a certain point—as far as I could go—and Steven didn't feel we had licked everything he wanted to lick, and he brought in Tony Kushner.

So, like Redford and The Horse Whisperer, *Spielberg had a vision, and you were partly depleted by the experience of trying to satisfy that vision.*

He wanted to feel that every possibility had been explored.

Did you come back and do any final writing on either of those projects— The Horse Whisperer *or* Munich?

No, I never returned to either of those.

So you never actually collaborated with Tony Kushner on Munich?

Kushner and I did not collaborate, ever. We never worked together, ever. I met him the night of the Golden Globes. Whatever was Tony's was Tony's and what was mine was mine. Some places they melded, and other places they didn't.

Do you feel the same type of frustration about Munich *as you do about* The Horse Whisperer?

I have the same feelings. There are wonderful things that are left of my work, and things that I wish had been included that weren't. There are things they invented that I didn't know anything about that are very good. And I could disagree with some of what they did. It's a director's medium—and a famous director like Steven, who has the kind of power he does, it's his decision what the movie is going to end up walking, talking, and looking like. All in all he made a very powerful movie.

And controversial.

A very powerful and controversial movie, and that's the reason to do those kinds of movies.

Thinking about it, maybe it goes back to why I didn't fight for credits earlier in my career. If I had worked on a movie like *Munich* in the '70s, if there had been a movie like that, with the same kind of power, maybe I would have wanted to share the credit. *Munich* isn't all mine and I can't take full credit for it, but I'm proud of *Munich*.

. . .

I'm surprised to learn that you wrote The Good Shepherd *after* Forrest Gump. *It had to wait more than a decade before it was made?*

I wrote it for Francis Coppola, originally. After *Forrest Gump* certain people asked me what I might want to write next and this was a subject I was really interested in: this monolith, the people who were in the CIA, the formation and early years of the agency.

Was Robert De Niro attached to the project early on, with Coppola?

No, later. Bob and I worked together for the last six to seven years on *The Good Shepherd.* I was doing other films, and so was he, but it was always a consuming project that was always part of us.

There were several other directors, earlier. Wayne Wang was on it, then Phil Kaufman, and John Frankenheimer before he passed away. John was the one who got Bob involved. John asked him to play a part in the movie. Bob read the material and loved it. When John passed away, Bob took it over. Bob had always been an aficionado of the CIA and even had his own project about the same subject matter, dealing with the later years of the agency. So we shook hands on making my movie, and I said if he would direct it I would write a part two for him later, which I always had in mind, if the first film worked. Actually I have a part two and part three in mind.

The second segment will be the one Bob was more interested in. He did become immersed in the first, obviously, and did, I think, a magnificent job. We became very close and still are and there is definitely going to be a part two—written; whether it gets made or not, we'll see.

Obviously you must have done a lot of research on this script. What books or people did you lean on the heaviest?

Many books. *The Cold Warrior,* the James Angleton book by Tom Mangold; *Old Boys,* by Charles McGarry; and *Mole Hunt,* by Nigel West. Books about Allen Dulles. And toward the end, I had the guidance of a wonderful man named Milt Bearden, who became our technical advisor. Milt had been a director of the C IA for thirty years and knew everything about the agency.

I wonder about certain literary touches in the script that probably aren't historical. The poetry scenes early in the story, or the miniature ship-building that is a hobby of Matt Damon's character. Where did these ideas come from?

The miniature shipbuilding comes from a friend of mine whose father was a CIA agent. The poetry was actually based on Angleton, who was a big aficionado of Ezra Pound.

What major changes did the script undergo over the course of those twelve years? Were you rewriting it constantly for the parade of directors?

The biggest change was structural, when Philip Kaufman had the material. Phil's an exceptional director. It was originally a linear piece and Phil changed it to nonlinear, so it would jump back and forth in time; it was an interesting approach and that stuck. With Bob it became more a matter of the refining of everything and finding out real details and having to make some tough editorial choices.

In order to pare the story down?

Pare it down and also make scenes more dramatic and find more truthful ways of doing things. Bob brought on Milt Bearden, who gave some verisimilitude to scenes that I couldn't have known about. So you learn more and the script grows. You could stay on one script forever without ever finishing it, especially when dealing with history and reality, but sooner or later, if you're lucky, you have to finish because they're ready to start shooting.

I have the same impression of De Niro as I have of Redford—not necessarily as a cautious person—but as someone who is meticulous and quiet and hard to read.

He's quiet, but I'm not sure he's hard to read *[laughs]*. He may be for people who are not close to him. He's very reserved and he's a guarded person, and he should be.

He's very specific in terms of script input?

He can be. He articulates when he needs to. He may not know the answer to how to do something, but he'll tell you what he thinks the scene needs, and from there it might grow into what it is. Hopefully, you'll find the answer together. In most cases, I think we did pretty good.

• • •

Let me just ask you briefly about Lucky You. *You are credited with the story as well as the co-screenplay. But you don't always get a story credit on films, even when you have contributed both the story and the script—in the case of* The Good Shepherd, *for example.*

You only get "story" credit if you end up "sharing" screenplay credit on a script based on your original story. There's no such thing as a "story-and-screenplay-by" credit anymore, as far as I know, so you only get a "script" credit if you end up finishing. If you get into a situation where somebody else does writing on your material, then they separate the credits, so that you can have the story credit. Whether you want it or not is a separate debate.

I had written that movie as an original many years ago for Warner Brothers—a love story set in Las Vegas in the world of poker. I had written it before the explosion of poker, which was then of no consequence in America, except for those who played it. Poker became widely popular, just coincidentally, after I'd written the script. My script was a somewhat stylish piece, rather humorous and tragic in its way. I thought it was rather beautifully done.

After I finished the script one of the executives sent it to Curtis Hanson and he signed on right away. He's certainly a qualified man and talented; he's done some good movies. We worked together on it for a while. It took three or four years for him to find the right actor, and then he opted to do another movie, *In Her Shoes* (2005), in between. Finally he got Eric Bana.

It wasn't the best working relationship for me, to be honest. Curtis always felt the need to, as he put it, run the script through his own typewriter, and he certainly had that opportunity. Again we had a different vision of the movie. This has nothing to do with the success or failure of it. The movie unfortunately didn't work, and sincerely I would have preferred that it had worked. It didn't work for various reasons, and I can't tell you what alchemy would have made it work. I think everybody tried hard, but the movie just didn't succeed.

Success and failure have a whole bunch of handmaidens. Obviously you're disappointed when you work hard on something and the public isn't attracted. But unless I were to direct a script myself, and I have no ambition to do that, it's never going to be right out of my mind.

That puts you in a very small category of top Hollywood writers who don't wish to direct.

I guess that's true. I don't think I'd be a very good director, is one reason. And I am good at what I do. So I'm always striving to write something that will be uniquely dramatized, and sometimes the films become slight disappointments like that, but nothing in a big way.

Which brings us to The Curious Case of Benjamin Button, *which is based on an F. Scott Fitzgerald short story and which, I gather, has been in the pipeline for years.*

I was the last of a long line of people, I guess. It has been in the works for twenty-five to thirty years. I was brought into it by Sherry Lansing, who thought, I guess because of my oddball-ironic look at life in *Forrest Gump*, that it might appeal to me. She also thought I might be able to write a nice love story, and I liked that notion too. The past versions by a number of writers hadn't found the light of day, so she gave me permission to do what I wanted with this great F. Scott Fitzgerald story about someone who grows old backwards. Kathleen Kennedy, as I've mentioned, was the producer of the project and she was very supportive. I just took off and wrote it.

It still took a number of years and some struggle to get the right director and cast. It was one of those scripts that didn't look like it was ever going to get made, to be honest. But it was also a story that resonated with people, and people loved my script and found it touching.

What unlocked the script for you that had blocked all those other people?

I don't know that I unlocked it, but it spoke to me. A lot of my stories have to do with the passage of time. I have a lot of children and grandchildren, and I'm fascinated by how age changes us and what certain remembered moments mean. I also like following the whole journey of a life, with people coming in and out of a person's life. With *Benjamin Button* I got a chance to look at the whole life of someone and also at the life of someone they love, whom they've grow up with. I got to explore the idea of what happens to people as they come together and grow apart.

Anyway the script finally landed in David Fincher's lap. He had known about the project for a number of years, from its other incarnations, and he had always loved the conceit of it.

Like Redford and Spielberg, Fincher doesn't do any actual writing?

No, but he does what a director should do. He's very smart, asks the right questions: "Why is this scene like this? How can we do it better? How can we make it shorter, or different, or mean more?"

Then the actors came on and read, Brad [Pitt] and Kate Blanchett particularly, and they had good, strong opinions, as actors should. I think we all worked very well together.

David, like Bob Zemeckis, is highly organized, and he didn't really need me after the script was done. When it was done it was done. A few questions popped up, and we conferred, or I changed something over the phone, or I went down on the set. Or he worked something out with the actors to make it comfortable for them and called me and said, "How do you like this?"

But unlike Bob Zemeckis, with David I've seen the dailies, which I have on my computer—I see what he shoots every day. Then, because he cuts almost simultaneously, he shows me cut footage in sequences and we talk about them too. The next step, once he's done, will be putting the special effects in, and he'll keep showing the film to me and I'll keep having opinions, and I'll be his eyes and ears to some positive extent when he needs me. I adore David, and from what I've seen he has made a very special movie. I hope I don't end up eating my words.

. . .

How do you choose from everything that is offered to you?

How do I choose things? Emotionally. I choose what I need to do at a given point, and sometimes I'm simply swayed by the prospect of a great adventure, and that I get to step into a world where you might not normally go, meet people you certainly wouldn't meet, and experience things you'd never get to experience. Some stories just excite me, some ideas, and sometimes when a studio calls and says, "How would you like to do this?" I say right away, "Sounds great."

It seems as though you never have writer's block or rarely take long vacations.

I work every day. I have no problem with that. I don't have writer's block very often. Any time I get nervous, or I can't fix something in a scene, I change the weather—so if it's "sunny," now it's "rainy"—and then I get a different point of view on the scene. I'm diligent about working, so every day I sit down and bang away at it. Generally something comes.

It may end up in the long run that it's not as good as I hoped it would be, but something does come. And on a day when I'm stymied I might just wrap it up. You live with it. You know you're going to live with it anyway.

Like recently I've been working on this script for Johnny Depp and it was gnawing at me—I wasn't sleeping. It's not like I got up at night to work at it. But it gnawed at me. Then, what usually happens is, I hear some sound, or see something, or feel something, and I get inspired. I go back to writing the script, and I push past the part that is gnawing at me. Maybe it isn't, for lack of a better word, to use a cliché, poetry. And that's what I want—poetry—something that sings. Maybe when I reread what I've written I won't feel that it really does sing, but at least I will have put down the rudiments of the idea and I might be able to go back and make it sing later.

I don't fight writing that way, where I have to get something absolutely right. Sometimes you have to slow things down. You can't feel pressured by what you're trying to put on the page. You have to take the perspective that it's not the end of the world if it isn't exactly right—move on—and then come back to it.

It sounds very practical.

Sometimes you have to get a little practical, even though as I say it eats at you until you feel like you've got it right.

You're very prolific. It sounds as though, quite apart from whatever new project you may be offered tomorrow, you have a dozen scripts in your drawer, or still circulating.

No. Maybe it would add up to a dozen, I don't know. The scripts that I have which aren't made—except for some very old ones that have gone by the wayside because time has passed them by—are a script I wrote about Dr. Richard Leakey, who saved the elephants in Africa. The "Commanche" script, which is still viable. "The Hatfield-McCoys," a script I wrote for Brad Pitt, which I still think will get done. Brad has been kind of busy lately, and part of his busyness has been with me—fortunately—on *Benjamin Button.* And I've just finished this "Shantaram" script for Johnny Depp, and I'm, at this moment, waiting to hear if Johnny likes it.

I'm keeping busy. I've just agreed to write *The Devil in the White City,* based on the best seller about events revolving around the 1893 Chicago World's Fair. And I've been given the go-ahead on part two of *The Good Shepherd,* so pretty soon I'll start on that.

November 2007

ERIC ROTH (1945–)

1970 I *Am Somebody* (Madeline Anderson). Co-director (documentary).
To Catch a Pebble (James F. Collier). Script.

1974 *The Nickel Ride* (Robert Mulligan). Script.

1975 *The Drowning Pool* (Stuart Rosenberg). Uncredited contribution.
One Flew over the Cuckoo's Nest (Milos Forman). Uncredited contribution.

1979	*The Concorde . . . Airport '79* (David Lowell Rich). Script.
	The Onion Field (Harold Becker). Uncredited contribution.
1981	*Wolfen* (Michael Wadleigh). Uncredited contribution.
1984	*The Pope of Greenwich Village* (Stuart Rosenberg). Uncredited contribution.
1987	*Suspect* (Peter Yates). Script.
1988	*Memories of Me* (Henry Winkler). Co-script.
1991	*Rhapsody in August* (Akira Kurosawa). "Special thanks."
1993	*Mr. Jones* (Mike Figgis). Story, co-script.
1994	*Forrest Gump* (Robert Zameckis). Script.
1995	*Apollo 13* (Ron Howard). Uncredited contribution.
1997	*The Postman* (Kevin Costner). Co-script.
1998	*The Horse Whisperer* (Robert Redford). Co-script.
1999	*The Insider* (Michael Mann). Co-script.
2000	*Chocolat* (Lasse Hallstrom). "Special thanks."
2001	*Ali* (Michael Mann). Co-script.
	Black Hawk Down (Ridley Scott). Uncredited contribution.
2002	*Frida* (Julie Taymor). "Special thanks."
2003	*Cold Mountain* (Anthony Minghella). "Special thanks."
	Duplex (Danny DeVito). "Special thanks."
2005	*Munich* (Steven Spielberg). Co-script.
2006	*The Good Shepherd* (Robert De Niro). Script.
2007	*Lucky You* (Curtis Hanson). Story, co-script.
2008	*The Curious Case of Benjamin Button* (David Fincher). Script.

Television credits include *Strangers in 7A* (1972 telefilm) and *Jane's House* (1994 telefilm).

Academy Award honors include the Oscar for Best Adapted Script for *Forrest Gump.* Best Script nominations include *Munich, The Insider,* and *The Curious Case of Benjamin Button.*

Writers Guild Awards include the Best Adapted Script for *Forrest Gump,* and Best Script nominations for *The Insider* and *The Curious Case of Benjamin Button.*

INTERVIEW BY **NICK DAWSON**

JOHN SAYLES THE NONCONFORMIST

If John Cassavetes is the father, then John Sayles is the godfather of American independent cinema, and has for more than twenty-five years been making intelligent, individualistic films outside the system. While Truffaut declared, "I make films that I would like to have seen when I was a young man," Sayles is a determined nonconformist who wants only to make movies that are unlike anything that has been made before; as he said in *Sayles on Sayles*, "Whether it is in the complexity that they're dealt with, or that I just feel like this is something that needs to be made."

In order to fund his distinctive visions, he has also worked as a Hollywood screenwriter and script doctor: in the 1980s he penned many more scripts for other people than he did for himself, and more recently it is through his uncredited work on major studio films that he has made much of his living.

Sayles was born in 1950 in Schenectady, New York, where he spent a childhood often cocooned off from the world. A quiet child, he read voraciously and, because of his insomnia, would listen to rock-and-roll radio stations and watch sports on TV through the night, often falling asleep in class the next day. He was a keen sportsman, but was overshadowed both in athletic and academic matters by his brother, who was a year older. Sayles's father's doctoral thesis on "the underachiever" was predominantly based on him, and despite going to college at Williams in 1968, he did not initially distinguish himself there. Having written and drawn since his early childhood, at college Sayles began to find his voice in writing classes, which he initially took to bump up his grades, getting involved in campus theater and discovering art-house films for the first time.

As was inevitable for a late-1960s college student, Sayles became politicized and went on antiwar marches, but avoided involvement in student political organizations, instead spending his spare time hitchhiking across the country, introducing himself to motorists as a different person each time. Through hitchhiking experiences, which included riding with Ku Klux Klan members and having drivers confess murders to him, he not only honed his storytelling skills but gained a greater understanding of America as a whole.

After his graduation from Williams, Sayles chose not to do a job that required further years of college, and so fell into doing blue-collar work and moving around the country. He worked as a hospital worker, did day labor, and sold his blood for money in Atlanta, then moved back east to work as a meat packer, writing all the time.

After numerous rejections of his short stories, an overlong short story sent to the Atlantic Press became his first novel, *Pride of the Bimbos* (1975). As writing did not pay the bills, while writing his second novel, *Union Dues,* published in 1977, Sayles worked as a carpenter's assistant and did summer stock theater with old friends from Williams. The cinematic style of his writing attracted Hollywood attention, and a move to the West Coast coincided with interest from Roger Corman's New World Pictures, which hired him to write the low-budget creature feature *Piranha* (1978). Sayles's love of genre movies made him an ideal Corman scribe, and he used the money he earned on *Piranha* and two other New World projects, *The Lady in Red* (1979) and *Battle beyond the Stars* (1980), to make his first feature. *The Return of the Secaucus Seven* (1980) was written in just a few weeks, shot in twenty-five days with his summer stock friends (including partner and producer Maggie Renzi), and released to great acclaim. Other screenplays Sayles had written around the same time—*Lianna* (1983), *Matewan* (1987), and *Eight Men Out* (1988)—would all make it to the screen over the course of the next decade, establishing Sayles as one of the most distinctive voices in American cinema.

In the 1990s, beginning with *City of Hope* (1991), he began to receive even greater and more mainstream recognition, with two of his films from this period, *Passion Fish* (1992) and *Lone Star* (1996), being nominated for Best Original Screenplay at the Academy Awards. The latter film, a portrait of life in a Texan border town, represents the zenith of Sayles's career thus far; it is a masterpiece, at once romance, murder mystery, and family saga, which deals with Sayles's continuing preoccupations of place, history, and race relations. Sayles has always been a political filmmaker, and his experiences while shooting *Sunshine State* (2002) in Florida led to *Silver City* (2004), an overtly political work released to coincide with the 2004 presidential election.

When I called him at his Los Angeles hotel (I was first put through to the sales department . . .) in the spring of 2006, he was trying to raise funding for his project "Honeydripper," about the roots of rock-and-roll. A few months later, Sayles wrote to me to say that the film, starring Danny Glover, was going into production that fall, financed totally by his screenplay earnings.

. . .

What kind of influence did your childhood in Schenectady, New York, and the Catholicism around you have on your writing—and your worldview?

It was Catholic in two ways. One is that Schenectady was a very mixed place. Certainly in the high school that I went to there were people of different ethnicities and religions and classes even, which is less and less true in public schools in the United States. But also I was raised as a Catholic, and one of the things about the Catholic Mass is that they read something from the Bible, from the New Testament almost always, and then there's a sermon about it. Even before I knew that there was a word for "metaphor" and "simile" and some of those other things that you use in literary fiction, I realized, "Oh, a parable! Something is like something." You'd hear these stories over and over every year. Pretty much on the same day, they'd read the same piece of the New Testament, so you'd hear about the fish and the loaves, or the wedding at Cana, or this or that or the other thing. And so those stories became familiar, and they're very allegorical, they have a lot of metaphors, they have a lot of similes in them, and sometimes the language is very beautiful.

What kind of films did you watch as a child?

I really did like all kinds of movies. I didn't see a foreign movie with subtitles until I was in college, so I didn't have an art-movie background. I would see some things that were dubbed. I remember liking [Vittorio De Sica's] *Two Women* (1960) when I saw it on TV, but it was dubbed into English. I really liked westerns, and later on I liked Kurosawa movies a lot, and Bergman movies, and started to see more world-cinema stuff. I liked film noirs a lot, but I certainly didn't grow up knowing who directors were, or barely even knowing that there were directors. It was "a John Wayne movie" or "a Gregory Peck movie" or "a Sophia Loren movie."

Did your early experiences working for Roger Corman help you to have that ability to get a movie started quick and cheap?

I think the great thing about working there was just that it was very practical. I wrote three movies, three movies got made. They had not chosen the directors when I wrote them, so I wrote the shots as if a computer was going to direct it, and then they would hire the directors after I was off the payroll. And then I'd get a panic call from the director, saying "There's no way . . . Do you know how little money he's giving me to shoot this epic of yours?!" So I'd usually do a draft off the cuff for them that was a practical one. And they had a little experience, those directors, they'd all directed at least one movie, I think, and we'd talk about the real practical thing of what costs money, and what doesn't.

Do you always have a stack of scripts ready to go, depending on what's practical for the moment? I know you wrote Lianna, The Return of the Secaucus Seven, Eight Men Out, *and* Matewan *in an intensive period in the late 1970s, and then had to wait a bit to get them all made.*

We kept trying to raise the money, and until we did we couldn't make 'em. I've got maybe three scripts right now that we could make, and we'll keep trying until we make them. But people get tired of you asking to finance the same project. Every once in a while you have to say, "Well, right now, we've run into a wall with this one. Let's try a different one." And there's a lot of luck involved.

With *Eight Men Out,* I think it finally got made because there were a lot of young male actors whom the studio—which had already turned us down twice—were interested in working with. Then the producers of it had just made a movie, their first feature for them, that had made a lot of money, and so the producers were all of sudden different people in the studio's eyes. I still don't especially think the studio loved the story of *Eight Men Out*—they would have liked it to have been more heroic, or whatever—but they were really interested in having a movie with all those young actors in it. So, sometimes just the climate changes, or your star rises, or the actor you wanted to be in it gets more famous, and so it's makeable.

You've written novels, short stories, you've developed a TV series, you do script doctoring, and you do your own scripts. Do you approach all these different styles of writing in the same way?

It's funny. I'm playing around with a novel right now. It's going to be a big novel, and it's going to have lots of characters in it. Certainly our movies have lots of characters in them and some different points of view, but in a novel you can be so much more "mosaic" than you can be in a movie, you can have so many more points of view—and you have so much more financial control. This is a period novel, so nobody would ever give me the money to make it as a movie. And it's going to be long enough that it's really about ten movies. So the ambition and scale that you can do in a novel, plus the scenes that you can cook up . . .

I always use the example in *Los Gusanos* [his 1991 novel], where I do, in seven or eight pages, the Bay of Pigs invasion. If I write in a novel, "The brigade walked down the road, their boots kicking up dust," they have boots. If we shoot a movie, the first thing the costumer does is ask, "Are we going to see their feet?" Because if we're not, she doesn't have to buy all those boots and make sure they're the right size. So it's a lot of money and work that we've saved. If I want it to be a hot, sunny day, which it was on the day that the brigade gets wiped out in my book, it's a hot, sunny day. If we're shooting a movie and it's raining, it's not a hot, sunny day! We either restage it for the rain—which is what we usually have to do, because we usually have a pretty fixed budget and time to shoot the movie—or we wait for a hot, sunny day, and just eat all that money that it took to get all those extras and airplanes and explosives and everybody else there. So there's that huge practical difference.

Also, it's weird, but the reviews I read when I first started out called the fiction writing that I was doing "cinematic." And then, later, because people knew I had written books, when I started making movies they'd say, "Oh, this is very literary," which it wasn't especially. But the particular type of fiction writing that I try to do actually doesn't include a whole lot of authorial comment. The story is usually what the people say and do, but the style in which it is written changes quite a bit according to whose point of view the story is in.

That seems to be something that goes through a lot of your work, that it's multiperspectival but your own perspective is not one of those included.

It's not included as a character's perspective, it's more like a lawyer presenting evidence. You don't present any evidence you don't want in front of the court, you do present the evidence that you need, but I try to do it just by putting the witnesses on the stand and letting them speak for themselves. I'm choosing the witnesses, however, and the order in which they show up. So there's quite a bit of authorial work, but I don't prefer to show my hand directly, you know. There's not a lot of "Dear reader . . ."

You can see how it varies with Faulkner, even. Some of his books are just people doing things and saying things, and he doesn't comment much on the story. And then other books are full of him commenting on things. In *Absalom, Absalom!* there's barely any conversation or dialogue in the book and not even that much action, but a lot of it is him going into the psychology and history of these characters. So even the same writer can use different strategies.

The strategy that I tend to use in most of my fiction is different from what you can do in a movie. An actor's going to play the character in a movie. I try to make all the people speak differently depending on who they are and how educated they are and where they're coming from, how old they are and what mood they're in. People can change, even within the same movie, but I don't have to show that within the text of the writing. And I don't have to give you a feeling that somebody's uneducated in the way that I might describe someone, because I know it will be done by the actors and the dialogue and through the point of view. So actually, there is a more "omniscient author" in my screenwriting than there usually is in my fiction writing.

The example I always like to use is, there's a Raymond Chandler short story where there's a line, "He gave me a drink of warm gin in a dirty glass." And from that one line, you get an idea of what the whole office looks like. Who would give you a drink of warm gin in a dirty glass? You know right away this is not a classy place. So if you can find that one detail, you don't have to do a half a page of description; the art department and the production designer are going to fill the rest in. But if you can give them that cue, that's great. That's a very omniscient cue, though it's almost like it comes from a technician working on the movie, not one of the characters seeing the action.

What we've been discussing touches on the conflict between your role as a writer and as an independent filmmaker, with what you write often having to be cut back because of budgetary restraints.

I think it's more that you have to censor yourself a little bit in your ambitions. I don't always. I've got a couple of really nice screenplays that who knows if we'll ever get to make them because they're very ambitious and nobody's been interested in financing them yet. Lately, it has not had to be very ambitious for it to be more expensive than anybody's willing to risk. If I had a $2 million movie, I probably could get it done right now, but who knows if I can raise any more than that. Our last movie *[Silver City]* we had to finance ourselves, and the last couple I've made were also down in the $2 million range, with somebody else paying for it. I would say it's definitely harder for me to sit down and, on spec for myself, write a very ambitious movie that would cost a lot of money, at my age now, than it was when I was twenty-five, when I had a lot of time ahead of me. *Eight Men*

Out I got to make eleven years after I wrote the script for it. Eleven years from now, I'll be sixty-seven. You just don't have that same feeling like you've got all the time in the world if you can't raise the money this year.

You have to be a little conscious of the business end, but I don't think you can let it rule you. Right now I'm likely to say, to start with, "OK, I've got a bunch of ideas for things to write that I'd like to make into a movie. What's one we can make really cheaply? Is there a unity of place? Is there a unity of time? Is it contemporary? Are there fewer characters?"—all those things that you know mean that you don't have to spend quite as much money. You might choose to put your energies into the cheaper one rather than something that might be a terrific story, and could make a terrific movie, but you're unlikely to be able to raise the money to make it. So it's that kind of self-censorship. And until I'm at the very end of a script, I tend not to do it. Once gone down the road where I've said, "I'm going to write this thing," I try to write it as well as I can. Then I may go back through it and say, "You know, trains cost an awful lot of money because of the insurance. Let's see if there's a way to transport them some other way than a train . . ."

I remember *The Untouchables* (1987), the Brian De Palma movie. They had a shoot-out on a train, and the insurance was going to cost so much that they restaged it—really pretty much at the last moment, after they'd already started shooting the movie—in a train station. Sometimes the cheaper way works just as well.

You used a train in Matewan, *I remember.*

On *Matewan,* we moved the train very, very little, and most of the shots are from outside the train. There happened to be a historical replica train going through the town, or coming near the town that we were in, and we convinced them to come through our town. It never had to back up, we got one shot as it pulled in. And then on *Eight Men Out,* we had a tiny little shot of a train pulling out of a station. It was such a short shot, and it was going to cost us so much to get a period train to move and maybe back up for a second take, that we actually built a platform that moved! We moved the platform forty yards *[laughs],* so it looked like the train was pulling out, made some steam and stuff like that, and it looks fine in the movie.

You seem to be inspired by place, and all your films are very much driven by the location they are set in, steeped in the history and personality of each place.

It certainly is an important part of the culture. If you see most Hollywood movies, where do they really take place? In Hollywoodland. Who would really own those clothes if that was their job? Who would have an apartment like that if they only make this much money? Where is it exactly? They're shot somewhere near Los Angeles, or they're shot in Toronto, and they pretend it's Chicago or Detroit or New York. So they aren't very specific to place or to culture, and that's not the point. The point of the movie is to be an entertainment that takes you away from anything that's real. It may be exaggerated to the point where it helps that it's not real.

The stuff that I do tends to be a little bit closer to recognizable human behavior, and that is influenced by where you live. People in Alaska live a different life than people in Alabama. The people in the Cajun part of Louisiana live a different life than the people in the Baptist part of Louisiana. New Orleans is New Orleans—there's nothin' like it. You're in New Orleans, you're not in any other Southern city. That specificity is something that interests me.

One thing that I've been able to do lately is, after one draft, go to the place and scout and decide where we want to shoot scenes and then start writing the subsequent drafts based partly on what we found there. Or sometimes I just have an outline of a story I want to tell—like with *Sunshine State* or *Casa de los Babys*—and I scout the place and see what's there, and then just incorporate the places so you don't have to build something. In both of those, for instance, there's a scene in a fort. One's an old Civil War fort, in the case of *Sunshine State,* and in *Casa de los Babys* there's an old Spanish fort. Well, I didn't build those, they were there. I said, "Jeez, they're there. How can I incorporate that into the action?" In the case of *Casa de los Babys,* I needed the poor neighborhood climbing up the sides of the mountains, and then a resort area and a hotel. And once I found those in Acapulco, then I started looking around for other things that were around there before I actually wrote the script. And it saved us a lot of money. There's a lot of production value that you get when you don't have to create something from scratch. It was only a four-week shoot, and we ended up living in the hotel where much of the story takes place for two weeks, so I had that great experience where you just roll out of bed and start directing! That means that you're not traveling during the day, so you get more shooting hours, and even that saves money.

But with Casa de los Babys, *it almost seemed like there was more of a story there than you had money to tell.*

In some ways that was, "What can I do now? What's a story that I can afford to make right now?" It was a story I'd had in my mind for a long time, and it was a very small, modest story. You could certainly extend it by having more of the other women's stories, but then it would become a TV series or a soap opera. It was designed to be a short film, a very low-budget film, a film that we could shoot in four weeks. So the ambitiousness of the film was planned; it wasn't something where I ran out of money or anything like that. Sometimes, if you want to continue as a movie maker, you have to say to yourself, "What's the least ambitious thing I have?"—at least in terms of money, not necessarily in terms of what the actors have to do, or whatever. Then, "Maybe that's what I should make now. Or what I have to make just to keep going."

The last time we spoke, which was a couple of years ago, you were trying to get funding for your project "Jamie MacGillivray."[1]

We've put "Jamie MacGillivray" aside for now. There just wasn't any interest in that project, and it didn't seem like the climate where anybody was going to be interested in it. I liked *The New World* (2005), Terry Malick's movie, but I don't think the fact that it didn't do especially well will help us raise money for "Jamie MacGillivray." To me, it's not similar at all, but in Hollywood terms, "Oh, it was an Indian movie and it didn't make any money at all." That kind of strange perception is more important than whether you get work, or people put money in your movies, or what actors are hot. Right now we're trying to raise money for a movie that I wrote a couple of years ago, called "Honeydripper." Last year, we missed out on our "window," because part of the story is set during the cotton harvest. You're locked into three months of the year when the cotton is high enough to harvest. It's about the roots of rock and roll, it's set in 1950, and we're still hoping to make it.

How easy is it for you when a film doesn't get made?

It's always disappointing, and it's more disappointing right on the day that you decide, "We're not going to get to do that this year." We had that moment with *Matewan,* when we were one day from flying to West Virginia to set up the office, and the people who said they were going to finance it called and said, "Oh, our bank loan didn't come through. We're not financing your movie." I said to the two producers at lunch, "Well, I have this other idea, and I've got $300,000 in the bank. Let's do it." They started "producing" before I had written one word of *Brother from*

Another Planet, and I think we were shooting six or seven weeks later. So sometimes you can throw yourself into something else.

But, you know, you do what you can. Like with this most recent one, "Honeydripper," last year we kept calling up crew members and cast people and saying, "OK, we're not going to start yet. We're going to push it back two more weeks, and if we can get the money, we can catch the middle of the cotton crop." Then we had to call again and say, "OK, they tell us that they can keep some cotton in the fields till this date, so we're gonna push it two more weeks." And you start to lose people, because you can't promise them you've got the money and they've got to make a living. So I think we went through three cinematographers. We didn't lose any of our actors, but we had to keep redoing the schedule. And then finally you have to make the call and just say, "We're not going to be able to do it this year," and you have to be responsible about that so people don't lose what jobs they could have gotten.

So, it's not an easy thing to do, and you lose money. We didn't lose a whole lot of money doing it, but you lose money. You've spent money on it, and sometimes you never get to make that particular movie, so the money is pretty much gone forever. Hollywood tends to spend a lot more money and then pull the plug at the last minute, and they may take a bath of a couple of million dollars sometimes.

• • •

How do you write? When, where, with a pen and paper, or on a laptop, et cetera?

You know, it depends on where I am. Right now, I'm on a trip to Los Angeles to talk to people I'm writing screenplays for, and I didn't feel like bringing my computer and lugging it around. I'm at the point where I'm doing preliminary stuff, so I just brought my notebook. Since I'm left-handed, I get notebooks that have the spirals on top, and I write. Usually, I won't do too many pages, no more than twenty, before I sit down and pretty much rewrite it as I put it into the computer. But, you know, if it was a different kind of trip I might have my computer and I might write directly into the computer. And I think pretty much with most screenwriters it's like having a certain amount of gas; if you have five weeks in which to do it, you do it in five weeks, and if you have eight weeks to do it in, you do it in eight weeks. And if you have two screenplays you are working on, you work . . . more.

So I write any time of day. I don't have to be at a desk; in fact I have problems with my back so I don't like to sit in the same place for too long.

I may write in three different locations in the same house in a day, or write some on an airplane, and some in the waiting room at the airport, and some in the hotel when I get there.

So there's not any real routine to it.

No, and then there's days when I don't get to write at all, or I don't want to write at all, or I'm doing research instead. I have a vague clock in my head of "I'd like to get this done in two weeks" or whatever, and it usually seems to get done.

I presume by this stage you know what are achievable goals, having been writing for so long.

Yeah, and with screenplays especially I tend to work up quite a detailed outline. Sometimes on an airplane coming back from a meeting I'll rough out the story and not write the scenes, but write, "OK, here's the location and here's what happens in the scene," and not bother with dialogue yet. Occasionally, if it's a rewrite, or something like that, and the structure is clear enough, if I have the computer with me I'll actually do all the scene headings, and even the shot headings, and then fill in the dialogue later. Things change, of course. Because structure is such an important part of screenwriting, I like to have a clear idea of it. So I rarely start without at least an idea of the structure. That sometimes is what measures your workday, not hours. You get to the end of a sequence that you know you're going to write, and you say, "Well, I've worked a long time today, I've worked enough today, and I'll start the next sequence tomorrow."

Are you in L.A. at the moment doing your own work, or doing script doctoring?

We're trying to raise money for "Honeydripper," which we want to shoot in Alabama, and so Maggie [Renzi] is up here and she's going around rattling the money tree for that. I'm meeting with Imagine, for whom I've been writing a screenplay based on an Italian movie called *La scorta* (1993), a Ricky Tognazzi movie from ten or twelve years ago that they want to remake on the Mexican border with the United States. I've got a couple of movies that I've just finished writing for people that are in their preproduction phase, which may be long, depending on actor availability or director availability. So you never know. I read about things that are getting made in *Variety*, just like everybody else. They don't call the writer up unless they need more work out of you.

Isn't "Jurassic Park 4" one of the scripts you've been working on?

Yeah. That was quite a while ago, and I did a couple of drafts on it. I don't know what their plans are. What I know is that the only purpose for making another one is that there's something different and cool that they can do. They don't want to just drag people back to the same island and have the same dinosaurs, or just a different species chase people around. And so I think the question they're struggling with is, "Is this new enough? Is this interesting enough to merit yet another one in the series?" You know, those movies are expensive, they're difficult to make, and yes, they make money, but why bother unless it's something new? And so I don't know where that script is at, or whether they've hired another writer, they're planning on doing it, or planning on not doing it. It was a full year ago that I worked on that.

Is your approach to writing a screenplay like "Jurassic Park 4" the same as it is on a film that you are planning to direct yourself?

Well, the main thing when you're working as a screenwriter for hire, you're helping other people tell their story. So I basically take the job if I feel like, "Well, jeez, there could be a movie made of this idea or this book that they want me to do, or this screenplay that they've already got that they want rewritten, which I could bring something useful to." There are some genres I'm just not interested in. I don't do slasher movies, for instance. And then, "Are the people reasonable? Have I worked with them before, and do I like them?"—that kind of stuff. You know, once you take the job, basically the first thing you do is ask a lot of questions. If it's a book, "What made you buy this book? What made you excited about it? What do you want to make sure to have in the film?" Or, if they've got a screenplay, usually they have twenty pages of notes of what they want to do with the screenplay; sometimes the notes are a little too general, but sometimes they're quite specific. I always liken the job to being a carpenter. You're not even the architect; you just come in and say, "OK, where do you want the windows?" So you use all the same muscles that you use when you are writing for yourself, and all the same skills, but you're helping them tell their story.

I was working for John Frankenheimer once and talking about doing a rewrite for him. He said, "Well, the drafts that have already been written are set in China, with Chinese people and Chinese martial arts. I can get Toshiro Mifune because I worked with him before on *Grand Prix*—let's make 'em all Japanese." And I had a week to do this rewrite because they were facing some strikes and other problems, and they needed to get a green light from a certain actor. I said, "Well, you know, the martial arts and the cultures are very, very different," and he said, "Yeah, yeah, I know. But I can get Toshiro."

This was on The Challenge*?*

Yeah. I said, "Fine, I can do that." Luckily, I knew something about those cultures and certainly about those martial arts, and I said, "It'll get better if I get to do a second draft of this, but in a week, I can change everybody from Chinese to Japanese. Chinese martial arts are circular and Japanese martial arts are much more back and forth, you know, straightforward. And there are huge differences in the cultures . . ." But I did it. If I had been writing my own script and I wanted to make something in China, the story would have stayed in China. But you're there to try and make their story good, you're not there to kidnap it and make it your story.

But there still has to be something that excites you, and something you feel you can add to the script.

Yeah. I like all kinds of movies. So I have to think, "Well, there could be a really cool movie that you could make out of this!" Occasionally I get to the point after several drafts where they're chickening out on what they first wanted to do, or changing their minds, and it becomes a movie that I wouldn't want to see. And that is usually when they get rid of you, or you get rid of them and just say, "Look, I don't think I can do a good job of where you want to go with this." But usually they've gotten rid of you much sooner than that. And occasionally I've done things where they've changed it radically halfway through the process, and I've felt like, "Yeah, you could make a good movie in that direction too!" and so I'm able to move there with them.

Because you have actors who regularly appear in your films, such as Joe Morton, Kris Kristoffersen, Chris Cooper, and David Strathairn, do you ever write with specific actors in mind?

You know, I try not to. You just never know if people, even if they're friends of yours, are going to be available or interested. So, I tend to write the characters, and then the first thing I think of is, "These are actors I like to work with, who can play this?" When I wrote *Casa de los Babys,* the only actors I'd had in mind when I wrote it were Rita Moreno and Vanessa Martinez, who I'd worked with a couple of times before. And the others, I just started calling actresses whose work I liked, most of whom I hadn't worked with before. So I don't—I try and write the character. And then you go through the script and say, "OK, this would be great for so-and-so, this would be great for so-and-so." And if they're actors you've worked with, you know how they work and things do go a lot faster.

With actors like Chris Cooper, though, people who've come through the ranks with you but now have a cachet in Hollywood, it must be easier for you with the studios to make a film with them on board.

You know that hasn't happened yet. I don't think that it's happened. I think sometimes investors have been mollified by the actors that we've cast, but we have to ask for the money before we necessarily have a cast. So we haven't had one I can think of where we got the actor to say yes, and people started running at us with money. I don't have anything against it if it's the right actor for the part, but that particular thing hasn't happened to us.

Does music influence you in your writing? In Silver City, *the music of the Cowboy Junkies seems a very important, almost subliminal presence.*

There was actually just one song in my head that I thought would work for a certain scene, and then I listened to that album *[The Trinity Session]* again, and I liked a couple of the other ones. You know, music in movies is such a trial-and-error thing. If you're using music that you've bought that you heard playing on the radio or whatever, sometimes you put it against the scene and it drags against it; sometimes the music overpowers the scene, sometimes the lyrics are too interesting, and the rhythm of the scene changes in a bad way. Every once in a while you put something there and you say, "OK, that's the right mood." And sometimes it's because it's unobtrusive but moody; sometimes it's because it's ironic when you play it against a scene.

I listened to a lot of things for *Silver City,* and that one song, when I stuck it in, worked, and then it turned out I liked the rest of the album and so I started trying some of the other ones. Unlike *Baby, It's You,* where actually I wrote the lyrics of the songs into the script and tried to get those songs, and got probably ninety percent of the songs that I had planned. I was thinking as I wrote, "OK, who does this guy listen to?"

Do you usually listen to music when you write?

Not especially. I'd rather just listen to music *(laughs),* and not be distracted by the writing. Actually, I'm not usually bothered by distractions. If I'm writing a screenplay and I'm sitting in an airport lobby and they're playing

CNN, it doesn't bother me that much. But listening to music does split my focus, and I'd just as soon write when I'm writing and listen to music when I'm listening to music.

So you weren't listening to border music when you were writing Lone Star*?*

Yeah, I was, but not literally when I was writing. Mason Daring—who's composed almost all of our movies—he and I will talk even before I'm writing sometimes, and talk about "OK, what's the music going to be like?" and "What's that genre? What are we going to do with it?" And then just try and steep ourselves in the genre. And that will give me sometimes rhythmic ideas or musical ideas, or I'll just learn more about the music.

For instance on *Matewan,* we listened to a lot of mountain music from the Kentucky and West Virginia region, and we finally just made the decision. "OK, we're gonna use all of this, except no banjo. This is not a banjo story." Some of that was because of the nature of the banjo, but some of it was also because for a general movie audience at that time, *Bonnie and Clyde* (1967) was still in their heads, along with all the movies that used banjo after *Bonnie and Clyde.* It's like you have to be very, very careful with the slide guitar now, or else it's going to sound like Ry Cooder did your score right after he did *Paris, Texas* (1984)—and like the millions of jeans commercials that have ripped him off. He was in a solid country blues tradition when he did *Paris, Texas,* but other people really liked the way it sounded so they did something a lot like it.

As you're in the relatively unusual position of being the editor as well as writer-director of your movies, do you ever end up having to cut out some of your favorite scenes?

Yeah, but I do that as a fiction writer too, though. David Lean cut some of his own movies; the Coen brothers cut their own movies—it's not that unusual, especially with independent filmmakers. But for me, editing is the third draft. You're still working with the actors and building the rhythm of their performances, and you're still telling the story.

With something like *Silver City,* we only lost maybe one and a half sequences, which was probably three minutes' worth of material, but almost none of the scenes are in the same order that they were written in or planned when we were shooting them. I got lucky. We had made the decision to have Danny Huston's character be a bit of a Hamlet, a bit of an outsider, a bit of a "I'm mourning for my own life" guy, so he's always wearing some kind of black shirt. And if you went back and looked at the movie, you would realize that his black shirt changes several times a day. So we were moving scenes with Danny in his black shirt, skipping twenty pages of script. The editing made the storytelling clearer, the "one thing leads to another" in his investigation a lot clearer. One of the reasons I find it's important for me to edit is I can't do the thinking involved in that unless I'm doing the editing myself. I can't have an editor do their version of the movie based on my notes, when I am still thinking about the final form. Just as I couldn't have somebody write a rough draft of a story and then have me finish it up based on their notes, and feel like I'd written it.

How loose are you when you're shooting? Do you rewrite on the set or allow your actors to do much improvisation?

You know, it would be nice to be a little looser, but we just don't do it. I can adlib better than a lot of people can write, and there's not that many actors that ad lib better than I can write. I certainly want the actors to stay with the text, but I also want to see where they can go with it. Marcia Gay Harden came to me when we were doing *Casa de los Babys* and said, "You know, this character is kind of a sociopath, there's just so many ways to play this," and I said, "I want to see them all." So if we did five takes, she did five very, very different versions of who that person was at that moment—because there was a lot of range within that character—but without changing a line.

I like to have the actors do the first couple of takes without changing a line, just to see what they're going to do with it, and sometimes what they do is not something I have thought of. And then adjust it. You know, a director doesn't teach anybody to act, or teach anybody how to do their job on a film set; you direct their talents. But for me, pretty much, the script is a given. I probably change three or four lines per movie. In the case of when people are speaking another language, and they speak it better than I do, we often talk about it. So like with some of the Mexicans and Mexican-Americans in *Silver City,* we talk about the lines and say, "How is this phrasing?" You know, my Spanish is learned, I didn't grow up with it. So I need to say, "For this character, how is this phrasing?" And then we'll sometimes adjust that. With the English, it pretty much stays the way it is.

How fluent are you when you're writing in Spanish?

Well, I can certainly write so anybody Spanish can understand what's going on, but usually I'll work with somebody who's a native speaker. On *Casa de los Babys* and *Men with Guns,* I had a Mexican friend go over the script, and then a Chilean guy, who's our boom operator, also read over it in order to tell me, "Oh, that's too Mexican!" I didn't want it to sound like it was Mexican—they were just Latin American countries—and I was trying to use a Spanish that would go for "generally South America" or "generally Latin America," without being that specific. After my Mexican friend had helped me with the dialogue, every once in a while there was something that they only say in Mexico, and the Chilean guy would say, "That's really Mexican. I've never heard that anywhere else in the world."

• • •

You are pretty much unique in that you play the Hollywood game to an extent, selling your services as a screenwriter, but you do that in order to get the money to make your own, very different films.

It's funny. You get typecast as a writer, or you get typecast as an actor, and there's no crossover. If you're an actor, they will indulge you and develop a movie that you want to direct, but it's pretty hard to actually get to direct that movie. You gotta be a pretty big star to have them just fork over a lot of money to direct your own movie. As a screenwriter, you're so compartmentalized. As I said, they don't even bother to call you when they're making the movie, or deciding to not make the movie. It just happens, or it doesn't. You read about it pretty far down the line. So, you're just not thought of as a director unless you're thought of as a director. So I don't get offers to direct things from Hollywood studios, and that's been a mutual understanding for a long time: what I do as a director doesn't especially interest them; and what they do, doesn't usually interest me as a director. The track record of our movies is such that some of them have been very successful on an independent level, but not on a studio level. They haven't made that $100 million that gets the studios really interested.

There's a quote in Silver City, *where it says that Danny believes that as a journalist he "should change things, not just report." As a very politically aware filmmaker, is this how you feel too?*

What I think is that journalists should try to tell the truth as best they know it, and that will automatically change things. The Reagan administration came up with this epithet of, "Oh, he's an advocacy journalist," basically meaning: "Anybody who disagrees with us or criticizes us is an advocacy journalist." But I don't think that a good journalist necessarily has to start out wanting to change anything; they just have to say, "Here's what I see is happening," and fight for the truth. Sometimes fight for the truth with their editors, in order to get it into the paper; fight to have it appear in one piece and not watered down to the point where it doesn't tell the truth anymore or is changed so it distorts the truth.

But I think mostly the guy who owns the paper sets the tone, and if he wants somebody to win as governor, he supports them, suppresses whatever is against the guy, and says whatever he needs to say to make the guy look good. He could be a good guy or a bad guy; it happens on both sides. This idea that there are journalists who call the shots is a fairly new one, and it's a nice idea, but it's very rarely the case.

I'm an advocacy journalist, in a way. I think if you tell the truth, sometimes people don't want to hear it and it's going to mess up their plans.

I mentioned doing something that changes things because Silver City *was released just before the 2004 election, and seemed specifically timed to have a political impact.*

Oh yeah. If you notice, you never meet the other candidate. You aren't given any opinion about the other candidate. It was meant to say, "Look at what's going on," while trying to be as honest as possible about what's going on. If people choose not to lie to themselves, or choose to ask a second question instead of accepting an easy answer or something that makes them feel good, that always automatically affects what's happening.

Finally, what lessons have you learned and how have you changed over your thirty years or so as a writer?

You know, I hope I know more about human beings *(laughs)*, and it's maybe some of the reason that the stuff that I do is getting even more complex. And probably one of the reasons that we have a hard time raising money to make the movies that I write. The characters are not necessarily heroic, and that's what Hollywood does very, very well and what audiences often really want to go to the movies for. So, we've chosen a rocky path to walk on.

April 2006

JOHN SAYLES (1950–)

1978 *Piranha* (Joe Dante). Co-story, script, actor.

1979 *The Lady in Red* (Lewis Teague). Script.

1980 *Alligator* (Lewis Teague). Co-story, script.

Battle beyond the Stars (Jimmy T. Murakami). Co-story, script.

Return of the Secaucus 7 (John Sayles). Director, editor, script, actor.

1981 *The Howling* (Joe Dante). Co-script, actor.

1982 *The Challenge* (John Frankenheimer). Co-script.

1983 *Lianna* (John Sayles). Director, editor, script, actor.
Baby, It's You (John Sayles). Director, script.
Enormous Changes at the Last Minute (Mira Bank, Ellen Hovde, Muffie Meyer). Co-script (anthology film).

1984 *The Brother from Another Planet* (John Sayles). Director, editor, script, actor.

1985 *Hard Choices* (Rick King). Actor.

1986 *The Clan of the Cave Bear* (Michael Chapman). Script.
Something Wild (Jonathan Demme). Actor.

1987 *Wild Thing* (Max Reid). Co-story, script.
Matewan (John Sayles). Director, script, actor.

1988 *Eight Men Out* (John Sayles). Director, script, actor.

1989 *Breaking In* (Bill Forsyth). Script.
La Fine della notte (Davide Ferrario). Actor.
Untamu giru (Go Takamine). Actor.

1990 *Little Vegas* (Perry Lang). Actor.

1991 *City of Hope* (John Sayles). Director, editor, script, actor.

1992 *Passion Fish* (John Sayles). Director, editor, script, actor.
Malcolm X (Spike Lee). Actor.
Straight Talk (Barnet Kellman). Actor.

1993 *Matinee* (Joe Dante). Actor.
My Life's in Turnaround (Eric Schaeffer, Donal Lardner Ward). Actor.

1994 *Men of War* (Perry Lang). Co-script.
The Secret of Roan Inish (John Sayles). Director, editor, script.

1996 *Lone Star* (John Sayles). Director, editor, script.

1997 *Men with Guns* (John Sayles). Director, editor, script.
Gridlock'd (Vondie Curtis-Hall). Actor.

1998 *The Newton Boys* (Richard Linklater). Song and lyric.

1999 *Limbo* (John Sayles). Director, editor, script, song, and lyric.

2000 *Girlfight* (Karyn Kusama). Executive producer, actor.

2002 *Sunshine State* (John Sayles). Director, editor, script, songs, and lyrics.

2003 *Casa de los Babys* (John Sayles). Director, editor, script, song, and lyric.

2004 *Silver City* (John Sayles). Director, editor, script.

2007 *Honeydripper* (John Sayles). Producer, director, editor, script, actor.

2008 *The Spiderwick Chronicles* (Mark Waters). Co-script.
The Toe Tactic (Emily Hubley). Voice actor (animation).

2009 *In the Electric Mist* (Bertrand Tavernier). Actor.

Music videos include *Bruce Springsteen: The Complete Video Anthology, 1978–2000* (director of "Born in the U.S.A.," "I'm On Fire," and "Glory Days," included in 2001 compilation).

Television includes *A Perfect Match* (script for 1980 telefilm); *Unnatural Causes* (script and actor in 1986 telefilm); *Shannon's Deal* (creator and writer of 1989–90 series); *Mathnet* (actor in series, 1991 episodes); *Square One TV* (actor in series, 1991 episodes); *Piranha* (co-story, 1995 TV remake).

Published works include *Union Dues; Pride of the Bimbos; The Anarchists Convention* (short story anthology); *Thinking in Pictures: The Making of the Movie* Matewan (nonfiction); *Los Gusanos;* and *Dillinger in Hollywood* (short story anthology).

Academy Award honors include nominations for Best Writing, Screenplay Written Directly for the Screen, for *Passion Fish* and *Lone Star.*

Writers Guild of America honors include the Ian McLellan Hunter Award in 2005, for lifetime achievement; and Best Script nominations for *Return of the Secaucus Seven, Passion Fish,* and *Lone Star.* Sayles's script for *Unnatural Causes* won a Best Television Script award from the WGA in 1986.

NOTE

1 "Jamie MacGillivray" is the working title of an eighteenth-century historical adventure, set partly in Scotland, that Sayles has been trying to launch into production since 2002.

INTERVIEW BY **VINCENT LOBRUTTO**

TOM STOPPARD ADVENTURES IN MOVIES

First, a little background. The man considered by many to be one of England's great living playwrights, screenwriters, BBC radio and television contributors, and masters of wordplay was born Tomáš Straussler in Zlin, Czechoslovakia in 1937.

Some (Sir) Tom Stoppard stats:

- The Stoppard clan moved to Singapore on March 15, 1939, when the Nazis decided to invade Zlin.
- Stoppard's father, Eugene Straussler, died at sea when his ship was attacked by Japanese forces (his mother would later remarry).
- Stoppard worked as a theater critic from time to time as a young man.
- Stoppard is known for his distinctive humorous writing style but also for his casual sense of couture and tonsorial fashion.
- The term *Stoppardian* refers partly to his wordplay but became part of the vernacular because of this writer's application of the droll and philosophical conceptual entity.
- Stoppard is a human rights activist. Some of the causes in which he has passionately involved himself include protecting the right to political dissent in Central and Eastern Europe, and the fight against psychiatric abuse.

This is how the interview transpired: Patrick McGilligan, who lives in the Midwest, came to New York for an appointment to interview Stoppard at Lincoln Center, where *The Coast of Utopia,* a monumental three-play cycle, was being mounted. Then fate struck. One of the principal actors fell ill and was not able to go on, throwing Stoppard and the company into a frenzied state. McGilligan's meeting with Stoppard had to be canceled.

A minibarrage of e-mails ensued between McGilligan and me, which concluded with my assignment to interview the formidable Mr. Stoppard while he was still in America and amenable. It struck me as ironic that a guy from Queens (the borough, that is), someone who has seen only a few plays throughout his life—two by Shakespeare, the rest by his favorite scribes, David Mamet, Edward Albee, and Sam Shepard—would get this daunting job.

I watched movies and read plays in a compressed time frame until I almost couldn't tell one from the other but was able to sort them out with clarity and focus due to Stoppard's distinctive vision of the world he lives and we live in.

Next, a series of phone calls sped up and down the phone wires, with Mr. Stoppard always being a gracious gentleman while I faked being calm, cool, and collected. When a date was set, I pushed on to a final prep and, on the day selected and agreed upon, packed my kit bag with tape recorder, McGilligan's questions, and my questions.

Here is what unfolded in the Upper West Side digs, where, one afternoon, Stoppard served me tea and biscuits and answered my questions, all the while delicately smoking Silk Cut cigarettes. (He of course asked me if I did as well—I don't—and if it would bother me; I said, "No, surely not.") My nerves calmed as I realized I didn't need to have two sets of questions clamped in my hand, and the Brit and the American bloke (with differences beyond mediums and country) found they had quite the bit in common. Let's listen in . . .

• • •

How did you become a writer? Were you immediately intrigued with literature, theater, and film, as a young man?

The first thing was journalism, not simply because I started as a junior reporter. When I was seventeen it occurred to me as a possible occupation. I knew or felt it would suit me instantly. I became a writer by becoming an ordinary young news reporter, and slowly got into feature and humorous writing until I got into pieces where I could use my own voice. I joined the newspaper in 1954, which was around the time the English theater began to become a hot spot in the culture. Thousands of men and women around my age began to think about writing a play.

I wrote my first play when I was twenty-three. Kenneth Tynan was at the *Observer*, Harold Hobson was on the *Sunday Times*, and the Royal

Court was the hottest theater in the English-speaking world. Then there was the French input. Samuel Beckett was a kind of French Irishman, and there were constant plays from Paris, plays by Eugène Ionesco and others. It all became very exciting. It seemed pretty wonderful at the time.

Wasn't that when the "Angry Young Man" films were coming to the cinema screens?

The Angry Young Man label came out of theater from *Look Back in Anger* by John Osborne. That generation got into films very quickly. Osborne, actor Albert Finney, and director Tony Richardson had a film company that made *Tom Jones* (1963), which set all three of them up for years to come. There were a lot young filmmakers making movies such as *The L-Shaped Room* (1962), and *This Sporting Life* (1963).

What were some of early film experiences you had that stimulated your imagination?

Next door to the newspaper I worked at when I was seventeen was the Gaumont Cinema. We worked all hours of the day or night so there was never any problem of going to the cinema in the afternoon if you were in between assignments. I remember seeing *Rock around the Clock* (1956), *The Ten Commandments* (1956), and *The Incredible Shrinking Man* (1957).The films which I absolutely adored would be *The Sweet Smell of Success* (1957), which is still a masterpiece, and *Some Like It Hot* (1959).

I'm a mainstream person with films. I never was one of those people who sought out exotic foreign films at some very small cinema on the side streets. I remember one Sunday afternoon Peter O'Toole and I went into a flea-bag revival theater in some suburb to see *Casablanca* (1942)—it was the first time I had seen *Casablanca.* Films of more recent history I absolutely revere would include *Chinatown* (1974). This week I saw *The Good Shepherd* (2006) and thought it was one of the best films I have seen in a long time. It's a grown-up movie; not every movie these days is a grown-up movie.

When did you write your first play?

In 1960. I was on a holiday in Capri hitchhiking around, and it was my twenty-third birthday. I had no money. I was eating a stuffed tomato watching rich people behind a great glass window being served by waiters. I sat there thinking, "I'm twenty-three today . . . , I'm behind schedule."

So I gave in my notice. I had no dependents and could live very, very cheaply. I retained a couple of weekly columns as a freelancer and sat down and wrote a play.

Many Americans have the impression that every person in England has some background knowledge about Shakespeare's plays. Did you have that kind of upbringing?

I went to a boarding school and we read Shakespeare. I wasn't taught in any inspiring way. They tended to read the plays in class. I gave an account once of Nerissa [Portia's servant] in *The Merchant of Venice.* At another school we were taken to see *Hamlet,* Laurence Olivier's production, for the good of our minds and souls—I was very bored by it. I much preferred a movie called *The First of the Few* (1942), which was about R. J. Mitchell, who designed the Spitfire *(laughs).*[1] When I was in my late teens I saw Olivier's *Richard the Third* (1955), which was a milestone for me and in my admiration of Shakespeare. I would still call it a great film.

What was your first film involvement?

The Romantic Englishwoman, which was a Joseph Losey movie from the Thomas Wiseman script based on his own novel. The producer was Danny Angel. He had two films that were ready to go. Losey was supposed to do whatever came first, and it turned out to be *The Romantic Englishwoman.* He was a man with a fascinating life. He spoke slowly and forcefully, and he was a sentient man. It was an interesting fate to find yourself working with Joe Losey.

Despair was even more interesting because it was directed by Werner Rainer Fassbinder. These adventures tend to be quite curtailed, because the writer is never around when the shooting is going on. I've had meetings with remarkable men, and then they go away and shoot the movie and I'm doing something else. So I met Fassbinder on only two or three occasions. Fassbinder was quite an alarming person. He was perfectly pleasant but I felt he was dangerous.

Despair is a novel by Vladimir Nabokov. It's about a man who encounters his own double, or believes it. I wrote the script assuming that Dirk Bogarde would be playing both roles, and I was surprised that Fassbinder and Dirk Bogarde certainly didn't want that. I may be maligning his memory, but I always had a strong feeling Bogarde didn't want to work twice as much. The film was made, and I was a real ingenue and imagined that one day on the screen would be the film I imagined. I saw a private screening and within a minute my heart was in my boots because I hadn't been on the set and the dialogue I had written which was to be played with ironic spin, seemed to be delivered with complete sincerity. The lesson for writers is they need a typeface for irony.

So on both of these projects you didn't sit down with the directors over long periods of time? You would get pages to the director, they would read it and get you notes?

Yes.

You weren't on either set at all?

No, and I seldom if ever give a director work-in-progress. I always wanted to get to the end of the script, let the director read it, and then see what he thought. When I was writing the screenplay for *Brazil* the director, Terry Gilliam, was a bit taken aback. He wanted to see what I was doing every two or three days and talk about it. I just couldn't work like that.

Could you talk about how you approached writing Brazil? *It doesn't take place in Brazil. It isn't about Brazil.*

Terry had a script, and it really didn't have any structure or narrative logic. It didn't really have any verbal humor. It certainly had humor and was full of wonderful writing, wonderful descriptions of dreams that were beautiful to read. He gave the script to me because he felt that it needed shaping into a narrative, and that pretty much was what my job was.

The moment I read it I began to worry that it would be taken as a kind of ripoff of *1984* and I started mumbling this anxiety to Terry. I said, "We must be careful to let the audience know that you're very well aware that *Brazil* is first cousin to the George Orwell book." Terry wouldn't engage in the conversation. Years later, he told me why, and the reason was he never read *1984*, had never seen the movie versions and knew nothing about it *[laughs]*![2] Something about the mythology of the novel trails behind it, but he really didn't know what *1984* was like and so he had no idea that Big Brother was in his movie.

In my interview with Brazil's *production designer, Norman Garwood, he talked about sitting in a room and somebody would come in with a hat with a shoe on it and say, "Is this it?" "Yes, that's* Brazil-*esque!"*[3]

That's Terry. Absolutely.

Did you see any of the sets, decoration, and props while you were writing?

No, I delivered the script. I went to a day's shoot just to say hello and there was such chaos. I never quite got a sense of what kind of movie Terry Gilliam was making. I like the film very much—it's one of his best films.

So the original script was by Gilliam and Charles McKeown?

No. Charles came in after me. They found some of my script too intellectual and then Charles came in to humanize it a little bit more.[4]

Have you worked with the novelist on any of your adapted screenplays.

No, I met Graham Greene twice thanks to Otto Preminger on *The Human Factor*. The sad thing is that Graham Greene was just one of a long list of really remarkable people who I met once or twice and never really encountered again or got to know them. I saw quite a bit of E. L. Doctorow before and during *Billy Bathgate*. I don't recall very much in the way of work happening. I'm sure we were talking about the script. I certainly wrote straight from the novel, as I did for example with *The Russia House*. I've been very fortunate in the novelists I've been privileged to interfere with: Greene, Doctorow, John LeCarré, and J. G. Ballard. It's a double-edged sword; perhaps one is slightly too in awe of the writer. I'm simply quite respectful. Temperamentally I'm a fan, and sometimes a novel needs to be disturbed more than my first draft.

Billy Bathgate was an unsatisfying experience, actually. I'm perfectly sure that Doctorow must have been very, very unsatisfied with the film. One of the curious things about making films is you rarely get on badly with somebody. Robert Benton is a particularly nice guy, there was never any problem on a personal level.

I came to New York once when they were casting *Billy Bathgate*, and in the office were all these photographs of young men . . . and Billy, as far as I can remember precisely, is a young teenager in the novel. He has an affair with the woman character played by Nicole Kidman. In the book he has the affair when he's fifteen years old. The whole dangerous edge of the book was that he was a child! I remember being shown a photograph of this young actor who looked as though he was twenty-one and was six-foot-two. I said, "But, but, but, but . . ." I felt out of my depth with these hugely experienced filmmaking people and didn't make a big song-and-dance over it, but looking back on *Billy Bathgate* it occurred to me that it went bad at that moment because Nicole was a young-looking woman, and there was no sense of a generation gap of any kind significantly between the boy and the woman he went to bed with.

I felt I had done some really good work. I spent a huge amount of time in the editing room afterwards. That's a phase of the process where I've been much more involved, literally, than in the production itself. I've always done that. That's where I've got to know the directors best. Stephen Frears has been a friend of mine since we did a BBC film together *[Three Men in a Boat]*, and that was because of the editing; the same with Michael Lindsay-Hogg, who did a television play of mine *[Professional Foul]*. I love being in the editing room because you can either save your film or make it fifty percent better, and I like to be there for that.

The film editor Carol Littleton called editing the final rewrite of a film.

I learned this from David Lean who said, "The hardest thing about shooting a film is to know at that moment how fast the actor should talk because it's something you cannot change."

You have to have a good ear in the theater; playwrights certainly have good ears.

In a way, being in preview with a play is not a lot unlike being in editing with a film. It's these adjustments in the rhythm and clarity—a lot to do with clarity. It's a thesis which I came to at some point, that the whole art of movies and in plays is in the control of the flow of information to the audience that's on the screen or the stage: how much information, when, how fast it comes. Certain things maybe have to be there three times. It's very, very much to do with letting the audience come and get what you want them to know. Don't withhold it an inch too much, because they won't quite get there and they lose concentration. Don't push it at them an inch too much forward, because then they lose the satisfaction of finding it themselves.

It's a continuous, fascinating preoccupation of the writer when the piece itself already exists, especially once you've had a preview audience at a movie or a play to respond to your sense of where the information is too much, or too little. That is the most fascinating and tantalizing part of the process, and there's no end to it. You can see that the stage performance is actually more exciting and more difficult, because you don't keep your gains necessarily. When you're cutting a movie, it stays the way you left it; theater doesn't.

Playwrights have a lot of control and should, over every comma, pause, and word. In the movies it's the opposite; you seem to take that pretty well.

That one I think broke his heart, it didn't do well at the box office. It's a sweet-natured film.

The emotional meaning of the film meant a lot to Steven, but when it came down to it people somehow did not care about it. Although it was well acted and well shot and everything, it didn't somehow reach where Steven wanted it to be—I don't know why.

Your principal collaboration with Spielberg was on Empire of the Sun, *based on the novel by J. G. Ballard. That is a great book and a tough movie.*

From the word go Steven knew which bit of it interested him.

As is well known, Steven's really attracted to a sort of father-son relationship, with a man and a young boy, and he was deeply self-aware about this. One of Steven's favorite films is *Captains Courageous* (1937). Ballard's book is like a wheel with quite a number of spokes, and there's no question about it that Steven responded to one of these spokes more than the others: the relationship between the [John] Malkovich character and the boy [played by Christian Bale] . . . though that doesn't really emerge until probably an hour into the movie. It is still a really good film but it's a very different film from the book. The first hour of *Empire of the Sun* is about as good as anything he's ever done; for me, it's wonderful. David Lean was going to do that film and Steven wanted him to do it, but he kept out of it until Lean said he was not going to do it. So Steven said, "Well, I've got to do it."

Any other Spielberg films that you have worked on?

I'm not sure what the rules are about these things because there are people's names on these movies, and I've done things which were really fun to do—very, very short-term things—but not all that much actually, very few.

But then they ring you up when you are naked and about to go into the bathtub.

Well, these things happen in different ways. As far as I remember about what I was told most of the time, I was asked to give a sort of lift to a scene, or to have some thoughts about the dialogue.

It's a widely known fact that very often there is almost no connection between the actual final script and the name of the writer credited with the film. Very often half or more of the movie is written by somebody else. Robert Towne is famous for it . . .

If I don't care more for some of the movies that I do it's because of the experience one has. I get excited about movies that I write. I say, "Yes! I want to do this one . . ." I get all excited and I tell people I'm doing it, and then maybe it gets into a newspaper that I'm doing it. I'm delighted, I'm glad I'm writing it. Then sometimes it turns out that the film made has absolutely nothing to do with you at all, and I feel sheepish about the whole thing. I must give you at least one example—I'm shooting my mouth off so much anyway—but I was fascinated by the Philip Pullman *His Dark Materials* trilogy. The first book was *The Golden Compass.* So I agreed to write a script.

I'm always optimistic about the situation. There was no director at the time. I was working directly for New Line, but the film is now being made by a very good guy, Chris Weitz, who loves to write his own scripts. He's never even read my script, which is okay, except it took up a year of my life, or most of a year, and in the end I said to myself, "I'm getting too old to throw away months of my life on something which is not going to happen." So now I've already begun telling directors, "I don't really want to, because there's no sense of security of it being 'my film' at the end. It will become another script by somebody else. I don't really have time for that any more."

Which one of your screenplays was filmed the closest to the way it was written?

Shakespeare in Love. John Madden had read what I had done. He liked it. He wanted to shoot it—he had some ideas to simplify it. I did get married to John Madden. I did have one director-husband, or wife as it were, because I really felt we were in step and he wasn't at all interested in changing anything. He wouldn't change even one word without talking to me. He conditioned the actors into the same attitude towards the spirit. I spent a long time with John, and the editor [David Gamble]—and subsequently with [producer] Harvey Weinstein on the telephone—so I was there right through to the end of the whole process, prior to the delivery of the film. When we were constructing or re-creating an ending for the film, to the last moment I was as much involved in that stage as it was possible to be. So that was the happiest film that I was involved in.

How did the story of Shakespeare in Love *originate?*

Marc Norman had the notion of a movie about young William Shakespeare in love, and it was his foundation—but they didn't shoot his script. What I did find in Marc's script was a good way in.

Have you ever written an original screenplay?

Never, I've never tried.

They become plays.

They become plays. I'm not sure why that is. I've never had an idea which said to me, "This has to be a film." I just think in a play form.

You strike me as someone who is a very disciplined writer.

I'm not so disciplined; I'm very disciplined when the crunch comes. I'm very, very disciplined then. I'll say, "Well, you can have this on August the first . . ." but in-between I'm rather casual.

I get asked to do a fair number of movies now. I might break off work on a play to diligently read this one or that one being offered.

Have you turned many film projects down?

Like any writer who gets things you turn down much, much, much, more than you do. Yes, of course.

What are the reasons? Is it that you just don't connect with it? You're not right for it?

I very often turn down a film project which I really enjoyed and liked reading. I turn down the adaptation job because it's not really what I like to do myself.

Even with plays there are all kinds of plays which I loved but they are not remotely connected with what I do myself. I turned something down this morning and something else a week ago. They are very different books, and they're both remarkable, one of them in particular, but I couldn't see where the movie was at all. Maybe there's a touch of laziness in this but there are certain jobs where you can sit down and start and get on with it; there are other jobs where you're going to spend three months reading and traveling and worrying because they are based on some historical source. It's a huge amount of time and work, and I just feel now, I'm sixty-nine—I'll be seventy this year—"Well, I really should stop doing what I've been doing, which is to read for three or four years, and then take two years to write *Arcadia* [his 1993 play]." I've spent a lot of time doing what's called "research," because I like doing research, and that certainly uses up your years.

One of your hallmarks as a writer is your use of wordplay. How does that interrelate with the visual aspects of a film?

I'm still hoping to learn how to write visually. I'm somebody who is approached by directors because they like what I write. Whether they ever say to themselves, "Well, Tom actually doesn't have a cinematic mind . . ." I have no idea. I'm still struggling very often to think cinematically. I think my scenes tend to be longer than modern cinema grammar is developing. I feel that I write movies as they did decades ago. I'm a verbal story teller, I'm aware of it, and if that's what somebody wants . . . though most of the time you end up feeling there are just too many words.

Tell me about the one film that you directed: Rosencrantz and Guildenstern Are Dead.

A producer called Michael Brandman had teamed up with a theater producer, Manny Azenberg, who produced me on Broadway many years ago. They wanted to make a film of *Rosencrantz and Guildenstern Are Dead,* and it was interesting because I remember making a list of twenty directors whose work I knew but more to the point that I liked personally. I kept looking at this list and I couldn't think of any reason why any of them should or shouldn't do it. All of them had made films that I'd liked, some I hadn't liked a lot, but they couldn't quite get the money for a film even as cheap as *Rosencrantz and Guildenstern Are Dead.* I don't know whether this surprises you or not, but it turned out that if I were to direct it myself the money was available.

The reasoning I worked out for that is that because I had never made a film at all, it was possible I'd turn out to be Orson Welles. There is something slightly sexy about the writer directing his own film. The other reason is very simple: I was the only director who could approach the material without undue reverence. I could throw material out, add scenes, I didn't have to worry about it being a so-called modern classic that people knew. I could just do whatever I liked with it.

The experience of making the film was in a less important sense horrendous, because one ends up on a telephone in Zagreb talking to someone in L.A. who promised some money . . . But in a primary way it was extremely inspiring and enjoyable. In an interview at the time I was asked about the experience of making the film and I remember saying, "I found it enjoyable," and I was rebuked for supposedly saying, "I found it easy." Well, of course I never found it easy.

You had a great crew.

Oh, you see the cleverest thing that I did was to get Peter Biziou to light it, and he brought in the production designer Vaughn Edwards, and they carried me. We did it in thirty-five days and of course I enjoyed the editing as I always do.[5] I filmed it in what was then Yugoslavia, with Gary Oldman and Tim Roth. The film was postponed for a year because of an actor's illness. Oldman and Tim Roth gave it a kind of modernity that was very good. It's not a great film, but I'll tell you one thing about it, if I could get it back I'd make it a few minutes shorter; it may be the only director's cut that would be shorter than the producer's cut.

Are you doing the next "Bourne" film?

No, I'm not. Another sad tale; no, it's not a sad story, I had a great time with the director Paul Greengrass. I had met Paul because of *The Bourne Identity* (2002). I'd turned down about twenty films. I'd written a play. I was waiting to come to New York to rehearse another play and I wanted to write a film while I was waiting. I love the Bourne films and I was talking to Kathleen Kennedy about something else entirely, and I said, "Well, who's writing Greengrass's film?" She said it was unclear and I said, "I would love do it, I love those films." Suddenly, I was writing *The Bourne Ultimatum* and I worked very hard indeed for three months, and then I had to go into rehearsal on the play. Paul is wonderful and he's also infuriating along the way, because he says it's wonderful one day and the next morning he says, "But suppose we did that . . . ?" And I have to say, "You can't just take that out and change that, it changes everything . . ."

So again there's a sense of one's pouring oneself into this script, which is then casually smashed one day, and you have to pull yourself into a slightly different one, and this was quite exhilarating while it lasted. Then I had to deliver the draft and go on and rehearse my play. Paul wanted me to come back, and I said, "Fine, I'll come back," but then the play was on and it was a while before I could say, "Well, I'm free again . . ." by which time everything had moved on. Later I was here rehearsing *The Coast of Utopia* and I tried to pop back on *Bourne* but the elevator doors closed again. About a couple of months ago Paul sent me the script and it made me laugh because I could see my molecules, but then I had to say, "I'm not going to do any more of your bloody films because I don't want to be the first of seven writers." I actually met the seventh writer—one of the writers lasted one day. It's kind of mad; they were still writing it while they were shooting it. But they pulled it off.

Now, wasn't there also talk about you doing a future Bond movie?

No, that was a sort of a joke; that was me talking to my agent and complaining about all these movies being offered to me about quantum mechanics or Jungian philosophy, and I said to him, "Why can't you get me the next James Bond movie?" A few weeks later, I read in the paper that I was writing the next James Bond movie and the press began asking about it—it was just a casual remark.

It's not that big a leap from some of the spy films that you've done.

I haven't seen the new James Bond [*Casino Royale*, 2006], but it needs to be different from the previous ones because one of the things that the Bourne movies did was to make the Bond movies look ridiculous.

Let's focus on your writing regimen. Is it different on a film script than on the plays?

No. When I am working, whether it's a film or a play, I work certainly to one A.M., maybe two or three. I go away from home with what I need—essentially pens, ink, paper, cigarettes, and instant coffee.

You work in an office or a writing room?

Until recently I had a house in France. I like somewhere where I can keep going. I like to work from noon until five and then pick up again about nine and then go into the morning—that would be my average day,

Are you sometimes working on two projects at once?

No.

Not a play and a movie?

I like movies *and* plays, but as I said before I've been a big cagey lately about films because I would just like to see one all the way through the shoot.

You have done a lot of your American film work in New York. Have you have worked in Hollywood very much?

It's quite a puzzling place. My experience is pretty much the same as everybody else's, which is that you get a sense the conversations aren't useful. The notes you get from the studios make your heart sink into your boots really. It's actually a curious and in some ways honorable phenomenon because every human being has a little flame, which says, "You too are as creative as anybody, you too are a creative spirit"—and the result is that people who are not really creative feel they can redeem their lives by influencing the creative artist. And they are not very good at it.

March 2007

TOM STOPPARD (1937–)

1970 *The Engagement* (Paul Joyce). Script (short film based on Stoppard's radio play).

1975 *The Romantic Englishwoman* (Joseph Losey). Co-script.

1978 *Despair* (Rainer Werner Fassbinder). Script.

1979 *The Human Factor* (Otto Preminger). Script.

1985 *Brazil* (Terry Gilliam). Co-script.

1987 *Empire of the Sun* (Steven Spielberg). Script.

1989 *Always* (Steven Spielberg). Uncredited contribution.

1990 *Rosencrantz and Guildenstern Are Dead* (Tom Stoppard). Director, script (based on his play).
The Russia House (Fred Schepisi). Script.

1991 *Billy Bathgate* (Robert Benton). Script.

1998 *Shakespeare in Love* (John Madden). Co-script.

2000 *Vatel* (Roland Joffé). English adaptation.

2001 *Enigma* (Michael Apted). Script.

2007 *The Bourne Ultimatum* (Paul Greengrass). Uncredited contribution.

2010 *Robin Hood* (Ridley Scott). Co-script.

Plays include *Rosencrantz and Guildenstern Are Dead; Enter a Free Man; The Real Inspector Hound; After Magritte; Jumpers; Artists Descending a Staircase; Born Yesterday; Travesties; Dirty Linen and New-Found-Land; Every Good Boy Deserves Favour; Night and Day; Dogg's Hamlet; Cahoot's Macbeth; Undiscovered Country; On the Razzle; The Real Thing; Rough Crossing; Dalliance; Hapgood; Arcadia; India Ink; The Invention of Love; The Coast of Utopia; Rock 'n' Roll; Henry IV.*

Radio credits include *The Dissolution of Dominic Boot* (1964); *"M" Is for Moon amongst Other Things* (1964); *If You're Glad I'll Be Frank* (1966); *Albert's Bridge* (1967); *Where Are They Now?* (1968); *The Dog It Was That Died* (1982); *In the Native State* (1991).

Television credits include *A Walk on the Water* (based on his play, 1963); *A Separate Peace* (1966); *Neutral Ground* (1968); *The Boundary* (1975);

Three Men in a Boat (1975); *Professional Foul* (1977); *The Dog It Was That Died* (based on his play, 1989); *Poodle Springs* (1998, HBO).

Academy Award honors include a Best Original Script nomination for *Brazil*, and sharing the Best Original Screenplay Oscar with Marc Norman for *Shakespeare in Love*.

Writers Guild honors include a Best Original Script nomination for *Brazil*.

NOTES

1 The Spitfire was the British single-seater that achieved renown as a fighter plane during the Battle of Britain.

2 There are two movie versions of *1984*, both British, made in 1956 and 1985. The earlier adaptation was directed by Michael Anderson and starred Edmond O'Brien, Michael Redgrave, and Jan Sterling. The 1985 version was directed by Michael Radford and starred William Hurt, Richard Burton, and Suzanna Hamilton.

3 Jim Acheson was the costume designer for *Brazil*. As Norman Garwood and the rest of the design team struggled to understand what look Terry Gilliam wanted for *Brazil*, Acheson came up with the concept of a "shoe hat," which he constructed and brought to Garwood, telling the production designer that he thought it was stupid. But in Garwood's view it was just what they needed to create the unique visual world of *Brazil*.

4 Terry Gilliam and Charles McKeown are also credited as writers of *Brazil*. McKeown's other credits include another Gilliam film, *The Adventures of Baron Munchausen* (1988), and *Ripley's Game* (2002).

5 The editor of *Rosencrantz and Guildenstern Are Dead* was Nicholas Gaster.

INTERVIEW BY **PATRICK McGILLIGAN**

BARBARA TURNER FREE SPIRIT

In Hollywood there is sometimes talk of the "short list" of top screenwriters, but one of the shortest in a film industry dominated by male executives is the list of women who have been getting their scripts produced for over forty years and who continue to work and excel at their job.

Barbara Turner was born in New York and started out her career as an actress in plays and television. She was married first to actor Vic Morrow and later to small-screen director Reza Badiyi, all three part of filmmaker Robert Altman's circle of friends and up-and-comers in the 1960s. Two of Turner's daughters are also actresses: Mina Badie (née Badiyi) has made many guest appearances on television series and played a lauded role in *The Anniversary Party* (2001), co-written and -directed by Alan Cumming and her sister Jennifer Jason Leigh. Jennifer is a familiar fixture in films; her numerous credits include a starring role in 2007's *Margot at the Wedding,* written and directed by her husband, Noah Baumbach.

Turner's niche is "troubled relationship" films, sometimes involving ordinary people, sometimes famous persons. The relationships are deeply troubled if not dead-end. Women are the focus of her empathy, with the plots usually secondary to a quirky, nonlinear structure.

Writing was initially a sideline, but more and more it paid the bills. Her Writers Guild–nominated script for *Petulia* (1968), a seminal 1960s film, established her unique voice. Yet Turner found more independence working in television and spent two decades writing acclaimed telefilms before roaring back in 1995 with *Georgia,* a brave, faceted gem that Turner wrote and produced as an independent starring vehicle for her daughter, Jason Leigh. *Georgia* concerns two sisters who have competed all their lives as siblings and musicians; one (played by Turner family friend Mare

Winningham) is a perfect success story, the other (Jason Leigh) an alcoholic loser. (A third Turner daughter, Carrie Ann Morrow, was a technical advisor for the film.) Roger Ebert was among the many critics who hailed *Georgia* as "a complex, deeply knowledgeable story abut how alcoholism and mental illness really are family diseases."

Since then, there have been several high-profile projects—*Pollock* (2000), with Ed Harris as the explosive abstract painter; and a reunion with Altman on the engaging ballet film *The Company* (2003). And the projects in the works make Turner's future look as intriguing as her past.

. . .

You started out as an actress. Why did you switch to writing?

It was an accident. Back when I was in New York in an acting class with Vic Morrow we were having trouble finding work, so we decided to write something we could shoot with parts in it for ourselves. We wrote an original screenplay about two deaf-mutes—so we could shoot it without sound—who come to New York from the country. That was the first thing we wrote, and it almost sold.

Then we came out here and we wrote a few other things. We wrote a musical together that we also tried to sell but it never got made. It was called "Willy Loved Everybody." It was very rural and very political. Elmer Bernstein read the script and agreed to do the music. He asked me to write the lyrics so that they didn't sound too professional. He thought they needed to be a bit clumsy. A sort of backhanded compliment, I suppose.

Had you any writing background before you became an actress?

No. School papers.

What is this first official credit of yours, the 1966 screen adaptation of Jean Genet's play Deathwatch, *directed by Vic Morrow? Was that more editing than writing?*

Yes. I trust the author generally when I work on a book or play. That film was very limited in scope, and it was staged like a play. Vic did a pretty good job working with pretty good actors.

You can't find that film anywhere to watch it nowadays.

I bet Paul Mazursky has a copy![1]

The first thing I wrote alone was "At Lake Lugano," based on a short story in the *New Yorker* by Mira Michal,[2] but I didn't know if I could actually adapt it so I wrote it first and then optioned the rights. It was about a young woman who'd been through a concentration camp as a child—now working as a U.N. interpreter in Geneva—and her difficulty with relationships. It takes place at Lake Lugano during a week's vacation with her lover. Anouk Aimée had agreed to play the part, Bob Altman was going to direct, and Columbia was going to make it. It fell apart, though, as these things often do.

I still like "Lugano" a lot. Every year someone reads it and says it should be made, and then we go through the hoops and eventually it doesn't. It really needs to be an independent film.

Anyway, Vic and I kept working regularly as actors, and one day I was working for Bob on some show, and he said, "You know, I have a book that reminds me of you, and you should read it. I think you can write it as a film." That was *Me and the Arch-Kook Petulia.*[3] I said, "I have no idea whether I can write it." He said, "I think you can," so I wrote it and it sold, and then I just kept getting work as a writer. It took me about three years to say I was a writer, however. I kept saying I was an actress for a long while, but I was earning my living as a writer.

Why did Altman say that about the book reminding him of you?

I guess Bob thought I was a free spirit.

For a long time Petulia *was going to be an Altman film, right?*

Yes, right.

Was he involved with the writing at all?

No. He was just letting me go. It was a very long script, the first draft was 190 pages. It's a funny story. When I showed it to him, Bob said, "Well, I'm going to send it out as it is. I'll just tell them that it's long." I said, "Bob, they'll know it's long. It's 190 pages." So what he did was go through the script and renumber it—18-A, -B, -C, -D, -E; 27-A, -B, -C, -D, -E—so then we turned it a script that was 124 pages. But it was really 190.

I still didn't think of myself as a writer. I wrote like an actress.

Can you explain that?

I write from the point of view of the character. I let the character guide me, moment to moment, as much as I can. I never start with an outline. I don't outline. I don't know how.

So you don't have a beginning, a middle, and an end in mind?

No. I do tons of research—tons and tons and tons—sometimes even as the picture is being made, I'm still doing research. And sometimes I'll have a thought for a last scene, but generally I'm not sure where I'm going until I see where the character takes me. I depend a lot on inspiration, sitting down and staying inside the character and letting the character take me. So the scene before dictates the next scene. I never say, "I don't know how to write this scene," and skip ahead and write the next one. I have to find my way there.

Anyway, I finished a draft of *Petulia,* but then Bob and his partner [producer Ray Wagner] split up, and in the split Bob got all the television properties and his partner got all the feature stuff. That was unfortunate. I continued with the project only up to a point.

Until Richard Lester came on . . . ?

That was not a good relationship.

Is there any way you can encapsulate the difference between Petulia *as a prospective Bob Altman film and how it turned out in Richard Lester's hands? Is it entirely a matter of style, or partly substance? Did the content shift?*

I think the content shifted too. And even though the script I wrote was nonlinear and the movie was, I believe, nonlinear, the script was more nonlinear. I think Bob's a braver director, more open. Dick Lester is very rigid.

I did one rewrite for Dick. When I first got to London, we had dinner and he said, "I can't wait for you to see the first draft." I said, thinking we were talking about the next draft I was going to write, "Neither can I." And he said, "Well, I'm giving it to you tonight!"

He had worked on it himself?

No, he had his friend—I forget what he called him—his "visual consultant," do a draft.[4] That's what Dick gave me to read, and you really couldn't make head or tails of anything in it, and it didn't have the American idiom.

I of course called Bob in a panic and flew back to L.A. overnight, met with Bob, who looked at what Dick had given me and agreed with me, got back on the plane, and flew back to London. We had meetings every day for a while. Dick said things to me like, "Your script is a vase [Turner pronounces it *vahz*], his script is a horse . . . and what we need is a something-something." I did what I could with the rewrite.

I couldn't see *Petulia* for a very long time, and when finally I did see the movie I could appreciate some of the stuff Dick did that was good, actually. The ending was different in the book and in my script, more romantic—a much more romantic ending—they [the George C. Scott and Julie Christie characters] ended up together. Dick gave it a tougher, more biting ending. I think that worked.

Did the unhappy experience of Petulia *have anything to do with your move away from feature films and into television writing? I'd think that because* Petulia *was such a high-profile success you'd have been inundated with other offers*

Well, I got some, but it just sort of happened that I ended up in television. I was hired to write a lot of film scripts that didn't get made, while the television stuff started getting made.

Was television a more hospitable environment?

Then? Yes. It was a momma-poppa store. You had just a few executives who were in charge of production, they had power, if they liked something it did not have to go to a committee. Now, it's all committee—thirty people have to give their notes. It wasn't like that, then. There weren't many notes, then, because the producers hired the people they trusted and they trusted the people they hired. They trusted the work.

Did it have anything to do with television being more receptive to female writers? There weren't that many women writers in features, then or now, really.

It's a nonpolitic thing to say but I never had that problem. Or I never thought of it as a problem—that I'm a woman writer. Just as I never thought of it as a problem that I was a woman actress. That's what I was, and I worked.

Was it the medium itself, and the kinds of shows as well as volume of work it offered?

It was that too. But the main thing is, the environment was different in television. It was a really creative environment. The people involved were creative. Four or five top executives, if you got to work with them, it was heaven. When they gave you notes, it wasn't for dumb-it-down viewing. When they gave you notes, it was about making something in the script work better, or clarifying something; not, "The audience'll never get it."

My experience with all the television executives I worked with—pretty much all, except later, when all television became a conglomerate and the MBA's started coming in—is it was a creative atmosphere.

I see that during those years, the 1970s and 1980s, you often wrote telefilms about relationships; often, difficult or tension-filled relationships—like Petulia. *How accidental was that, or did it grow out of* Petulia?

I guess it did come out of *Petulia* and possibly "At Lake Lugano." Relationships are always exciting. They're like lightning in a bottle—certain kinds of relationships—something explosive is always around the corner. People struggling to connect with each other and themselves, to find out who they are and where they fit in this world: it's the human comedy, and something we all relate to on some level. We've all been there, or are there.

I like to quote from Andrew Sarris's interview with Ingmar Bergman from his book *Interviews with Directors.* I used to read it before I started every script. It touched and inspired me deeply and still does.

At one point Bergman says: "I am sometimes asked what I am looking for in my films, what is my goal. The question is difficult and dangerous, and I usually reply with a lie or an evasion: 'I am trying to say the truth about the human condition, the truth as I see it.' This response usually satisfies them, and I often ask myself why nobody notices my bluff, because the real response should be: 'I feel an irrepressible need to express in film that which, completely subjectively, is part of my consciousness. In this case I have therefore no other goal but myself, my daily bread, the amusement and respect of the public, a sort of truth that I find to be right at that particular moment.' And if I try to sum up my second response, the final formula is not very enthusiastic: 'An activity of no great importance.' "

The part where he says, "And we finally run into a dead end where we argue with each other on the subject of our solitude, without any of us listening to the others or even noticing that we have pressed so close to one another as almost to die of suffocation," especially resonated with me. Anyway, it's a long interview, ending with, "A little part of myself will survive in the anonymous and triumphant totality. A dragon or a demon, or perhaps a saint, it doesn't matter," but he says things much, much better than I can say. Certainly that interview was one of the main influences on my writing.

Petulia*—and some of the telefilms—are about relationships that are also touched by some sort of illness, mental or physical. Why is that?*

I guess that's true, although it's hard for me to think of it that way. Aren't we all touched by illness?

Were you often writing directly for the performers, or the strengths of a certain performer, in television—knowing in advance who the stars of a particular telefilm were going to be.

No, I never did that, even though sometimes I did know who was going to play the part. Even with *Georgia,* which I wrote specifically for Jennifer and Mare, it always became about the character.

When you wrote the 1973 telefilm The Affair *for Natalie Wood and Robert Wagner, you weren't thinking of them all the time?*[5] *They weren't, in a sense, hovering over your shoulder?*

No, they weren't, because I wrote that script before I met them. Once you get into the material, it has to be about the guys on the page.

Do you write differently if it's a script for television or film?

No.

Not even in terms of budget?

Sometimes, because I would always rather work for an independent [company], like with *Georgia,* because independents leave you alone.

When you were working so steadily for television in the '70s and '80s were you also trying scripts occasionally for film projects?

I must have written some. There were a lot of scripts I was employed and paid to write that didn't get made.

Isn't that a depressing aspect of the job?

For a while. Because you've had the experience of the work you'd like to see it reach some fruition. But you get over it.

And if you're lucky, you've gotten paid.

I've been very lucky in that regard, though it isn't all about the money.

. . .

What brought you back to feature filmmaking with Georgia?

Jennifer said to me, "I have an idea for a movie we can make." She was working on a film where she played an undercover drug cop [*Rush,* 1991], so I flew down to her location in Texas. She told me this idea for two sisters—one of whom Mare [Winningham] could play—one who has talent, the other one doesn't.

Okay, Jennifer's your daughter, but why Mare?

My eldest daughter, Carrie Morrow, when she was sixteen, ran away and joined a carnival. A very close friend of the family, a producer, Phil Mandelker, knew the story and thought it would make a great script for television. So I wrote that script; it was called *Freedom*, and the producer got Mare, who at the time was a pretty big TV name, for the part. She came over to the house to meet me and said, "I would like to stay with your family for a while and see what it's like living with you." So she moved in for about a month before the filming and then stayed here all during the shoot.

Prior to that, Mare and Jennifer had gone to an acting camp together (they're about four years apart in age). So Mare was like an extended member of our family.

So it started with Jennifer's idea? Had she written anything down?

No.

Where did you go from there?

I started with, "Where should we set it?" Actually I wanted to set it in Austin, because of its music scene, and it was Jennifer who said, "No, let's go to Washington." So I went to Seattle and hung out with bands for about three weeks initially, me and my assistant.

Were you doing the whole thing on spec?

All on spec, although Jennifer paid me to write the script, which included expenses for the trip to Seattle and a research assistant. It took three years to get it made. We got [director] Ulu [Grosbard] very fast once the script was done, and he'd read it. Then we got French money.[6]

How long did the actual writing take?

After the research . . . about a month.

Is that standard for you, or faster than usual?

Once I start to write, it's 24-7—it's the research period that takes more time.

Is it really 24-7?

The last couple of days it's sixteen hours days. Before that, I just keep writing until I dry up, hit a wall.

There's so much music in the story. Was all of that specifically detailed in the script?

Yes. I had a great assistant, and she kept bringing in music for me to hear. I kept listening and listening, because music is so important to *Georgia*. Music is really part of the dialogue.

Do you generally listen to music anyway while you are writing?

If I'm going to put it in the scene, maybe. Sometimes I'll stop and search for a piece of music for a scene. Or I'll remember a piece that I think is right, and put it in the script.

I mean, do you use music for inspiration, to set a mood for yourself?

Not always. I watch a lot of movies.

As a break from the work?

I watch movies for inspiration. Like [Krzysztof] Kieślowski—I think he's a god—I forget what movie I was writing, but I watched *Red, White,* and *Blue* over and over again.[7] The visuals are so rich, and for me what the camera is seeing gets me into a scene. If I don't know what I'm looking at, I can't write the scene. I have to know what I'm looking at.

Do you include a lot of description of characters and settings in your scripts?

Yes! Endless, endless. I remember I gave a talk to a film class once, and one of the students told me, "In our first class the teacher showed us a sample from *Georgia* . . ."—of course I was flattered to hear this—" . . . and he told us *never* to do that sort of thing!" Because the first page and a half has no dialogue, it's all description, and it will go into the oval file; no one will read it. I said, "What can I tell you? It got made."

Is it camera description or literary description?

Both.

Do you write endless dialogue as well?

Sometimes I'm sparse, sometimes it's too much. I always think less is more, but then on the biographical scripts I tend to want to use everything these people said so the script fills up with talking scenes.

I'm told you have a unique quirk when writing dialogue—that you often eschew question marks.

Yes, because I don't think people speak in question marks. "Where are you going." Not, "*Where* are you going?" So I either don't hear it in my head as a question mark, or even though it's a question I hear it like a statement. "What time is it." Not, "*What* time is it?" If I mean something to sound like a question mark, I put in a question mark. Otherwise I leave it out.

When you are writing characters, as much as possible are you drawing on real people?

Yes.

People you know intimately?

Sometimes. But Jennifer is not playing herself in *Georgia,* she is playing somebody else who is real. She draws on herself, of course. The great thing about writing for Jennifer, and Mare too, but especially Jennifer, is that there is no place she can't go because there is no place she won't go. She's so fearless that it's very freeing.

In Mare's case there's a lot of Mare in that character. Mare has five kids, and I went and lived with her family for two weeks, even though I'd known her for a long time. I picked up little bits and pieces—the way she cooks, how the household operated.[8]

Georgia is full of stories that came from the musicians that I met. I just gave the stories to the character that was appropriate. These were all semi-failed musicians in Seattle; they'd been around doing covers mostly, but they were still doing it. I hung out with a lot of them, and borrowed something from all of them.

Is the realness of the characters important to you?

Yes, even if they're fictional characters. If I'm going to write about a lawyer, I have to go spend a day—at least a day—at a law office.

Georgia*—and many of your stories—revolve around people's problems, their conflicts, their pain.*

Yes, I like complications.

Because there's more inherent drama in the situation?

No, because it's stuff you connect with.

Once Ulu Grosbard was on board as director, did he recommend any changes in your script?

No. He shot the first draft practically. He would not let anyone change a word. An actor auditioning asked if he could improve the dialogue. Ulu said the dialogue had its own music and rhythms and couldn't be changed. After the audition I thanked him. His response was, "I didn't do this for you." If it ain't broke, he doesn't fix it. As producer, I was on the set every day. It was thrilling. It made for a dream experience.

• • •

After Georgia, *you directed a short film, according to IMDb.com.*

I wish. It was called "A Beautiful View" and it wasn't a short script; it was supposed to be a feature that Jennifer was going to be in—a thriller. It would have been a lot of fun.

Is there any chance it will be revived?

Every year it comes up. Every year two things come up—"At Lake Lugano" and "A Beautiful View."

Let's talk about Altman and The Company. *How did you get involved?*

Neve [Campbell] came to me through her agent. She of course had been a ballet dancer and had a deal with Warner Brothers to do a ballet movie. There was a script done which she didn't like, she thought it was "too Hollywood." She wanted it to be more like the reality. She met with me because she had liked *Georgia,* and then I didn't hear from her for about two years. She meanwhile abandoned the Warner Brothers project and then, when she came back to me, she said, "I want to start from scratch." I said, "Why don't we try and do this sort of like a Mike Leigh film—but not quite; that is, we should just go live with the Joffrey Ballet for a year and build the characters that way." That's basically what happened, although she couldn't live with the company all that time, so she'd drop in from time and time and dance with them. I'd stay with them for a couple of weeks, go away, and then come back and stay for another couple of weeks.

Everything went on tape. I'd just sit and talk with the dancers, in groups, and one-on-one. Then I wrote the script, and it was about the company. I got it to Bob and told him, "I think you're the only person who could understand this movie." He said, "This is an area that interests me a lot," and he agreed to direct it.

Had you stayed in touch with him over the years?

Not really, not a lot, but he was working with Jennifer during that period.[9] I called his office pretty much out of the blue and said, "I would love you to read this." *[Growling Altman imitation:]* "Of course I'd read anything you wrote."

That brought you full circle back to a director you had worked with forty years earlier. How was your collaboration this time?

We fought a lot. Screaming fights. Mostly he screamed. I just talked back. A lot of it became his, as all things do with Bob. It became a "Bob film."

Other than *Petulia* (which was a tremendous experience), I had worked with Bob mainly as an actress before. He loves actors and actresses. They can do no wrong. Writers? Ehh!?

It was a wholly different relationship, and what I had expected was the acting relationship and the *Petulia* relationship which we'd had, which was glorious. But still . . . if you have an opportunity to work with Bob, you work with Bob.

In the beginning I brought him tape after tape of the company doing ballets, and we'd sit and watch the tapes together and talk. We had this running disagreement. Before I knew there would be any problems, Bob said, "This movie is about dance." And I said, "This script is about dancers." He'd say, "No, this is about dance," and I'd say, "No Bob, this is about the dancers, it's about a company of dancers." "No, it's about dance." You wouldn't think that's a big difference, but it is. His movie was more about dance than it was about the dancers in an odd way, drawing a really fine line.

He is great to work with, though he drives you crazy. There's a story I tell: He said to me, "I love your script, but this is your script and now it will have to become my movie." "Oh obviously, Bob," said I. Then as we got closer and closer to filming, he said, "Listen, what is important to you is important to me. The script is long, we have to cut some stuff. So I want you to write down the ten scenes that are most important to you." I did. He didn't shoot one of them. I realized that is what he meant by, "This is your script but it's got to be my movie."

There was one scene, for example, that I thought was essential—the end of the movie. *The Company* was the first time actually that I knew how I was going to end a movie before I started the script, because I had a painful, extraordinary ending in mind. The ending was the auditions for the ballet company, two hundred people crowded into a room that is very warm—102 degrees—young dancers being dropped every few minutes—some very talented, some not. That is where I wanted to end the movie, with the company auditioning for ten openings the next year.

And he cut that too?

Yes.

The film needs a better ending.

There are many things like that I miss. And all along Bob came up with bits of business that he put in, a lot of funny stuff.

But the script and film are really very similar. Many of the relationships are similar. The main thing is Bob wouldn't let the dancers—even though it was their dialogue, I didn't invent it—he wouldn't let them see the script. I had had actors read it to them several months before the shoot, so that they knew I hadn't betrayed their trust. He'd say, "You come in here in this scene and say something like . . . " The actors needed the script, so they had the script, and said pretty much what I wrote. The scene structure pretty much went untouched. And the film was beautiful and pretty much critically well received. But the dialogue of the dancers changed.

Bob is so tricky. For example, despite our disagreements, he wanted me on the set all the time. *[Growling Altman imitation:]* "Turner! . . . Where's Turner?" Which was funny, because sometimes I would be happy to be on the set, watching, sometimes I would be shattered.

Then why'd he want you there?

I don't know. Because that's Bob. I had been on the set with my scripts before. Even on many of the television shows I wrote, I was on the set. This time . . .

At the first formal screening Bob asked, "Well, how did you like your movie?" I said, "It's your movie, Bob." And we bandied that back and forth for several minutes.

But as angry as you can get at Bob, it's impossible not to adore him. We were going to work on something else together—something a group of us were trying to get done as a special television event, based on a book called *But Beautiful,* by Geoff Dyer, about jazz musicians. We were going to get a different director for each musician, and Bob had said yes.

It took me forever to accept the fact that he had died.[10] I kept thinking it was a mistake, and that he would reappear. He seemed incapable of dying.

. . .

How did Pollock *originate?*

A very young producer—twenty-one at the time—first talked to me. He sent me this seven trillion page book about Pollock. I knew nothing about Pollock, but I fell in love with him. The young producer had gotten the rights to the book and went into a partnership with [actor] Ed Harris. They called me and interviewed me over the phone. They asked me what I would do with the subject. I said I would write the script like one of Pollock's paintings—it'll go backwards and forwards and sideways; each scene will propel the next in terms of storytelling. And that is how I wrote the original first draft. Nonlinear.

Several years went by. There were other directors before Ed. The fact that *Pollock* got made I really lay at Ed's feet. He pushed and worked, pushed and worked.

Meanwhile I cut and cut the script. It was indecently long. And eventually, when Ed ended up directing the film, the nonlinear aspect had to go, because Ed felt he needed more structure.

I think he did a great job. Especially the painting sequences, which I thought were great, and the relationship sequences with Marcia [Gay Harden, who plays Pollock's artist-wife Lee Krasner] were super. And it's a beautiful picture. But there was a lot about the other painters that was in the original script. The approach was a little more epic in my script, covering that period in art. Ed skimmed out anything that was nonessential. I was sorry to see that and the nonlinear thing go.

It sounds like so many years and so much work, on these projects. When you saw Pollock *eventually, was it like watching a movie where you see parts of it that are distinctly yours—and other parts that are like viewing your script through a funhouse mirror?*

It's really hard the first time. I had to take someone with me to look at *Pollock* because I didn't think I could judge it fairly. And that was the truth—after the first screening, I didn't know what I was seeing. My mind was so clouded, with stuff going through my head, that I couldn't judge it fairly. Then I went to all the festivals with it, and saw it a lot and thought about it a lot, and I began to see the film for what it is. So it took me a while to really see it.

What's next for you? What script of yours looks most likely to be filmed? Is it this "Ernest Hemingway Project" that has been mentioned in the trade papers?

That seems to be crawling forward now. It was really moving rapidly ahead for a while, before it fell into development hell. That's with [actor] Jim Gandolfini and [director] Philip Kaufman. It's about the relationship between Hemingway and Martha Gelhorn.[11] That relationship was really a combative one.

Once again it seems you have been drawn to an incredibly fractious relationship.

I was always fascinated by Martha Gelhorn, actually, and by that relationship. I've always thought Hemingway was a piece of work. She was an amazing journalist, much better than he was, even though he got her into it and made her a journalist. When she writes an article you feel like you're there. When he writes an article, it's about Hemingway. "I did this, and I did this, and I did this . . . " But she puts you there. Their relationship was very fraught, because he wanted to be nurtured and she wanted to work. She wanted to be where the action was, and he was sick of war.

Their story should be told as it really was, because nothing is more fantastic in this case than the truth. It was an exciting and brilliant and battering relationship. They knew how to speak and could cut each other to pieces with words. They did and said things that are hard to believe. It would be a shame to fictionalize that.

Did you work closely with Phil Kaufman? Did he do any writing?

He hasn't written anything yet, but who knows?

My dream is to work with one independent after another, because otherwise the work loses some purity—it has to—unless your production unit is somehow strong enough to fend off HBO, or MGM, or whatever. When you work with the major companies, it's often endless dumb notes. I do my best to work with them, but I'm not very gracious when confronted with dumb notes. I bristle and talk back and say, "No . . . are you out of your mind?!" I say it as graciously and as collaboratively as I can, but I'm not very good at it.

June 2008

BARBARA TURNER (1936–)

1966 *Deathwatch* (Vic Morrow). Script.
1968 *Petulia* (Richard Lester). Adaptation.
1995 *Georgia* (Ulu Grosbard). Producer, script.
2000 *Pollock* (Ed Harris). Script.
2003 *The Company* (Robert Altman). Co-story, script.

Television includes *The Affair* (1973 telefilm); *Widow* (1976 telefilm); *The Dark Side of Innocence* (1976 telefilm); *The War Between the Tates* (Emmy-nominated adaptation for the 1977 telefilm); *Freedom* (1981 telefilm);

Sessions (producer and writer of 1983 telefilm); *Eye on the Sparrow* (producer and writer of 1987 telefilm); and *Out of the Darkness* (1994 telefilm).

Writers Guild honors include a Best Script nomination for *Petulia.*

NOTES

1 Future writer-director Paul Mazursky (see *Backstory 4*) headed the cast of *Deathwatch,* which includes Michael Forest, Gavin McLeod, and Leonard Nimoy.

2 Mira Michal, "At Lake Lugano," *New Yorker,* August 15, 1964.

3 John Haase's novel *Me and the Arch-Kook Petulia,* published in 1966, explores the relationship between a divorcing San Francisco physician (played in the film by George C. Scott) and a quirky socialite (Julie Christie) battling inner demons and an abusive husband (Richard Chamberlain).

4 David Hicks was credited as the "design consultant" on *Petulia.*

5 *The Affair* is a love story between a crippled songwriter (played by Natalie Wood) and an older lawyer (Robert Wagner).

6 *Georgia* was funded by the French production company CiBy 2000.

7 Acclaimed Polish filmmaker Krzysztof Kieslowski capped his career with *Trois couleurs: Bleu* (1993), *Blanc* (1994), and *Rouge* (1994), before his untimely death in 1996.

8 Mare Winningham was nominated for an Oscar for Best Supporting Actress for *Georgia,* and Jennifer Jason Leigh won the New York Film Critics Circle award for Best Actress in the film.

9 Jennifer Jason Leigh played pivotal roles in the Altman films *Short Cuts* (1993) and *Kansas City* (1996).

10 Altman died in November 2006 of complications from leukemia. He finished only one more film after *The Company: A Prairie Home Companion,* released the same year as his death.

11 Martha Gelhorn (1908–98) was a novelist, travel writer, journalist, and war correspondent who was also the third wife of Ernest Hemingway. They divorced in 1945 after four acrimonious years of marriage.

I take it pretty well because I do have theater. If I had only movies I'd probably be much more frustrated about it all, but you know, you go in there knowing what the score is, and what the rules are.

Generally speaking, I enjoy doing the first draft of the screenplay as I enjoy writing a play for the stage, and maybe even the second draft. If it goes beyond that, then the climate changes and progressively you become the tool of the true author. It can get tiring. You lose the energy which comes from your own creativity.

There are situations where a writer and a director get married, and they're a team, and they're much more a part of the process than in the films I've been involved with. Joe Losey got married to Harold Pinter for a few years, and they were a writer-director partnership. I've been involved in movies where I've been brought in and they've got a problem and they've already had three writers, and probably three more after me as well. Well, it's one way to make a movie, but you see why somebody who has another life on the stage doesn't take it all that seriously, when these movie adventures occur.

What was it like to work with Steven Spielberg?

He's so good at making films, so in the end every film is well made, but to him it matters whether it was good *before* it was made.

How did he relate to you as a writer?

I've had very interesting times entering and leaving Steven's life for a short period or a longer period. I like him very much, we get along well, and I consider him a friend. When I was trying to prepare my own film I'd talk to him and he was generous with his time. Steven is somebody who's likely to call me in the middle of a production and say, "Listen, can I send you a couple of pages? There's something I . . . "

I remember once he was making a movie and he phoned up and he said, "I need this, and the guy who wrote it has gone away." This fax arrived as I was about to have a bath, and in this house I lived in then I had a study which happened to be next to the bathroom with a connecting door. I had no clothes on and I was standing there stark naked looking at these two pages, and I thought, "Oh, I see . . . " So I picked up a pencil and wrote him a couple of pages which went into the movie. I like to think that those few bits of film were written by a man who was stark naked.

What film was it for?

It was just a fragment—like a page or two at the most—on *Always.*

INTERVIEW BY **LEE HILL**

RUDY WURLITZER QUESTING

Roads that turn in on themselves or go nowhere, frontiers coming to a close, and characters seeking meaning on the fringes—these are all constants in Rudy Wurlitzer's work as a novelist and screenwriter.

A similar questing and restlessness can be found in Wurlitzer's life. Born in Cincinnati in 1930, Wurlitzer, like William S. Burroughs, was heir to a once prosperous entrepreneurial dynasty known for its player pianos and organs. He spent most of his childhood and youth in New York, where he studied the violin. When he became a teen, he embraced the Beat ethos of wandering for its own sake. From the mid-1950s through most of the 1960s, Wurlitzer moved in and out of various emerging countercultural scenes in the United States and Europe to the extent that time and money permitted.

His first novel, *Nog,* published in 1969, didn't sell very well, but its mix of the mythic and the avant-garde caught the attention of Monte Hellman, who hired Wurlitzer to completely rewrite Will Corry's draft of *Two-Lane Blacktop* (1971). The result was so startling that Wurlitzer's screenplay was published in *Esquire,* and *Two-Lane Blacktop* was hailed on the magazine's cover as the "film of the year" months before its release. Unfortunately the film, with its quasi-Beckettian take on the conflict between two young hot-rodders (played with stone-faced brilliance by James Taylor and Dennis Wilson) and an older, enigmatic long-distance driver (Warren Oates, delivering a performance both avuncular and sinister), went over the heads of the post–*Easy Rider* audience Universal hoped it would pull in. Over the years however, the film has come to be seen as a great lost masterpiece of the 1970s New Hollywood era.

Two more uncompromising novels, *Flats* and *Quake,* appeared in the 1970s. Neither sold particularly well, but their cryptic storylines found favor among mavericks like Hal Ashby and Sam Peckinpah. Wurlitzer's collaboration with Peckinpah on *Pat Garrett and Billy the Kid* (1973) was a more thoughtful and compassionate take on outlaws trying to escape their past than *The Wild Bunch* (1969). Although the film was cut heavily by MGM, the current director's cut on DVD demonstrates how well suited Wurlitzer was to bringing out the best in maverick sensibilities.

By the late 1970s, after several promising projects were trapped in development hell and work as a script doctor became less appealing, Wurlitzer retreated to Cape Breton, New Brunswick, where he worked with Robert Frank on two experimental films and the independent feature *Candy Mountain* (1987). Since then, Wurlitzer has worked almost exclusively outside Los Angeles with directors based in Europe, most notably Alex Cox on *Walker* (1987); Ridley Scott on a pre–David Lynch version of *Dune;* Michelangelo Antonioni on "Two Telegrams" (which surfaced in abbreviated form in *Beyond the Clouds*); and Volker Schlondorff on *Voyager / Homo Faber* (1991). While some of these collaborations, such as his work on Bernardo Bertolucci's *Little Buddha* (1992) and Carroll Ballard's *Wind* (1992), were not completely successful, Wurlitzer preferred the less corporate style of collaboration embraced by non-Hollywood directors. Wurlitzer has also continued to write books, most notably the memoir *Hard Travel to Sacred Places* (1991), and the novels *Slow Fade* (1984), inspired by his experiences with Sam Peckinpah, and *The Drop Edge of Yonder* (2008).[1]

Although on many occasions he has come face-to-face with the mainstream studio development process at its most dispiriting, Wurlitzer talks about screenwriting with a healthy blend of idealism, patience, enthusiasm, and stoicism. He has not only managed to work regularly with directors who shared his open-ended approach to narrative, genre, and character; he continues to refresh himself with new books and collaborations on operas with old friends like the composer Philip Glass.

This interview was conducted by telephone and e-mail in the spring and early summer of 2008.

• • •

EARLY YEARS

I was born in Cincinnati, but my mother and father moved to New York, and I spent my most of my early childhood in Manhattan. When I was quite young, I played the violin. My father at the time was a dealer in rare stringed instruments so I played the violin up until my late teens. Then I grew more obsessed with literature, writing, poetry, jazz, and drugs.

I started traveling at a very early age. When I was seventeen, I worked on an oil tanker and went to the Persian Gulf, and one of my first short stories came from that experience; that sense of adventure has become more complex as I have gotten older. I attended Columbia for four years, then I went to Paris and sat in on lectures at the Sorbonne, and then I went to Aix-en-Provence and attended a few classes at the university there. I also went to Harvard briefly for a couple of summers. My academic background is mostly English literature and philosophy.

I met the composer Philip Glass in Paris. He was there spending time working with Nadia Boulanger. Philip and I were both pursuing the same girl, which neither of us was successful at *[laughs]*.

Later in New York, in the '60s, we became close friends. He was working as a plumber and I was just trying to survive. One summer we went up to Cape Breton, Nova Scotia. By then he was married with kids, and we were both pretty broke, so we shared a house. We ended up buying a property there that we divided, and we would go up there off and on through the years. I have been up there for a few winters over the last thirty-five years or so. That was where I also met Robert Frank, who lived about twenty miles from us.

LITERARY INFLUENCES

My first short stories were naturalistic, but I became very influenced in Paris by Samuel Beckett, Celine, E.M. Cioran, among others, and to a lesser extent the French *nouveau roman*. In New York during the late' '50s and early '60s, there was a ferment of creative activity. I did some happenings with Robert Rauschenberg and Claes Oldenberg and even made a little film on Oldenberg. Philip and Steve Reich were doing music. There were jazz people such as Charlie Parker, Ornette Coleman, Cecil Taylor, Thelonious Monk, John Coltrane, and Charles Mingus; writers like William Burroughs, Allen Ginsberg, Ken Kesey, Frank O'Hara, and Jack Kerouac. These different kinds of expressions were very stimulating for me in New York in the '60s and '70s, full of radical cultural surprises and romantic permissions.

The first thing I had published was a short story, "The Octopus," in the *Paris Review*, and then another, "The Boiler Room," in the *Atlantic Monthly*. In 1969, I published my first novel, *Nog*. In and around that period, to pay for the privilege of writing obscure books, I began working in film, and that represented a sort of livelihood rhythm, which began a pattern of alternating a piece of prose every couple of years or so with a script.

Film has always been a big influence and I have always been obsessed with the great filmmakers, especially the Europeans like Godard, Truffaut, the Russians, Akira Kurosawa, Ingmar Bergman, and all kinds of other people, as well as filmmakers in the States like Billy Wilder and John Ford. I was a film addict. But I got into writing scripts because I was a friend of Jim McBride's.

Glen and Randa was the first script I did with McBride, whom I knew socially in New York along with Lorenzo Mans, a creative collaborator of Jim's. After *David Holzman's Diary* (1967), Jim went out to California to do *Glenn and Randa.* I came out to California, excited to help Lorenzo and Jim with the screenplay, a form I had never written in before. Because the film was so independent and unencumbered by commerce, everything with Jim felt free and open-ended.

MONTE HELLMAN AND *TWO-LANE BLACKTOP*

After *Nog* was published, Monte Hellman was looking for a writer to rewrite this script, *Two-Lane Blacktop,* by Will Corry. Monte liked my *Nog* a lot and called me up and asked if I would work on Corry's script. I totally rewrote the whole script. I didn't take much of Corry's script, except the names of the characters—the Driver, the Girl, and the Mechanic—and the idea of a cross-country race in a hot rod, but I couldn't use any of the other stuff because Corry's work was very conventional. When I told Monte I couldn't use any of Corry's—I would have if I could, but it wasn't where I was at—he said, "Great, do what you want to do!" which is pretty unusual. I think I was able to write in such a free way at the time because Monte Hellman gave me total permission.

There were no meetings about the script, and luckily I didn't know much about writing screenplays. I was completely free to explore that form in an open-ended way. I wrote the script quite fast . . . thinking about the idea of road and what it means to be on the road. It wasn't going to be about winning or losing. Or going from *A* to *B*. It became a very interesting exercise especially since I didn't know much about cars *[laughs]*.

I did hang out in San Fernando Valley with a lot of car freaks and read a lot of car magazines and sort of embedded myself in that world. It's funny because after the film came out, it showed in this little theater in Cape Breton and these guys from the town would come out in these modified cars and lift up the hood and ask "What do you think?" and I didn't know what they were asking me. I lost a lot of face up there *[laughs]*.

It was amazing that the complete screenplay was published in *Esquire*. I am not sure how it got to *Esquire* . . . probably my agent sent it to them. The publication had its ironies because *Esquire* called the script the "film of the year," and then, when the film was released, they said it was the "flop of the year." *Two-Lane* didn't exactly do well because the film was so existential and went against the genre of the racing movie. It didn't incorporate traditional ideas about car racing, as well as user-friendly character development that involved a beginning, middle, and end. It was a film that pushed a lot of buttons, and in fact was panned wildly by many critics. It is only recently that it has been re-released on DVD through Criterion; it has been given another life and become a cult film of sorts.

In the end the journey in *Two-Lane* was more about process, being in the present, the road for its own sake inside an existential and alienated cultural envelope with essentially no past and no future—frustrating stuff for a film audience used to who wins and who loses. These days, now that *Two-Lane* has become part of "the '70s," one is aware that the whole nature of aimless travel and being on the "road" has changed. Given the current state of things, with fuel, cars, travel, freedom, exploration, film is a more philosophical and melancholy experience. It's also a funnier film now, given its obsession with the unconscious, somewhat adolescent attachment to the myths of freedom and journeys and relationships that lead nowhere in particular.

As a director and collaborator, Monte Hellman is a gentle gifted purist who has managed to survive outside the commercial grid of Hollywood. Monte enters scenes first through his eyes, then finds a way to deal with whatever a character might be demanding. In this way, he sticks to a script, which is always satisfying for a humble scribbler. He's strangely innocent and unpretentious, which often leads him into uncharted and surprisingly original waters.

SAM PECKINPAH AND *PAT GARRETT AND BILLY THE KID*

While I was out in L.A. a producer, Gordon Carroll, asked me if I would like to do a western and so I got involved with this script, *Pat Garrett and Billy the Kid,* and they asked Peckinpah to direct it.

That production was even crazier than what you read *[laughs]*. There were lots of moments. At one point, someone from the studio came down to view a screening of dailies. Sam was completely confrontational with him. It was a ferocious evening, and from then on it was very polarized between the studio and Sam, but Sam fed on confrontation. That tension fueled and united everybody in terms of the cast and crew.

One thing that stands out is that there was an actor who was supposed to play the little part that I played, who went back to L.A. suddenly, so I got to play the part. When it came time for me to run out of this shack and get shot, Sam did about thirty takes and he kept saying over and over, "I just love to shoot writers!" *[laughs]*.

I got burned out and left before the very end of filming, but I remember the production very fondly because of that old outlaw-all-the-way-to-the-end point of view that Peckinpah had which would never be allowed now. Working with Sam was unforgettable, he was one of a kind: ornery, charming, perverse, dangerously defiant, and skillful.

It was a different time in the '60s and '70s, the atmosphere was much more spontaneous and loose. It wasn't so hierarchical. I also worked on several projects with Hal Ashby, which unfortunately didn't work out, although I did the last rewrite on *Coming Home.* We spent a lot of time together and were good friends.

People like Peckinpah and Ashby were mavericks in their way, as well as such people as Bob Rafelson and Jack Nicholson . . . ; there was a sense of benign anarchy among certain individuals in Hollywood at the time . . . ; it was great to be there and I really liked being in the West. From L.A. I made a lot of journeys to remote parts of the western U.S. and I really liked that part of it as well.

Where the corruption starts is just doing it for money. How attached you became to shaking that particular money tree is where the corruption begins—no one is asking or forcing you to do it, it is self-imposed corruption. People get hooked and attached to the whole commercial monocultural glitz, but I don't blame Hollywood for that; that is just what Hollywood is. It is up to the individual to make his choice.

As films became more and more expensive, with a global outreach, they also became more and more reductive, so the language of film became more and more sublimated to image and the dictates of megabudgets. It really became out of balance. In the '30s and '40s, there were wonderful writers, who had their own hard times, who came out of the New York theater, and whose language had a totally different meaning in the context of the collaborative film medium. I'm sort of related to that tradition a bit. I like language, I'm obsessed with language and the inventiveness of playing with words, so I had to leave Hollywood in order to pursue that in earnest.

ROBERT FRANK AND *CANDY MOUNTAIN*

After my stints in L.A., in the late '60s, early '70s, I bought my place in Cape Breton with Philip Glass and his wife. Cape Breton was sort of a very off-the-grid place where I could go to recover. Robert Frank lived up there too, as he still does, and we became very close friends and started working together in a spontaneous way; that was another rhythm, so to speak, of making films. And one way of working helped the other, personally, so that after working on a Hollywood script I'd find myself drawn into this other domain . . . and it became another kind of exploration in terms of language and finding out what I was really thinking about.

Most of what I have done is about exploring various kinds of frontiers. I am a very nomadic character. I travel a lot and have lived in different places, but it is not just geographical and historical frontiers that I have been involved in, but spiritual, psychological, and internal frontiers as well. I would say frontiers are on a certain level my broad overall subject.

I did three films with Frank, two shorts: *Keep Busy* and *Energy and How to Get It*, besides *Candy Mountain*. He helped me recover from the monocultural toxicity of Hollywood, and he offered a free-floating process of discovery and adventure for its own sake. We never knew where the script was going, everything was completely spontaneous, almost to a fault. Robert was like an action painter, improvising, always in the present, sometimes dangerous, often difficult, defiant about preserving his integrity, often stubborn, take-no-prisoners, always unforgettable, even nourishing. In our short films I placed myself in the middle of the action, writing and conducting a through-line as we went along, and in that sense those were true collaborations.

Even though *Candy Mountain* was a low-road independent film it was the largest one Robert had ever been involved with, and for me it was a good experience only up to a point. I felt very free in terms of the script. The mistake is that I co-directed; it rarely works to have a co-director. Ultimately the only way we could direct together was for me to let Robert do it his way. So I fell back and just tried to survive. He always respected and followed the script, so that part worked well, and I did do a lot of things on the film. But it was sort of psychologically complicated, and our relationship suffered and, sadly, was never the same. I don't have bad feelings about the film or him, but it was difficult, and I would never co-direct with anyone again. I just don't think it works. It is like having two prime ministers.

For the most part there is a very complicated relationship between the writer, the director, and the producer and the money element, with the writer more or less sublimated to the process; you don't really have the authority you would have writing a book—the autonomy. Psychologically, writing films is a much more perilous occupation; that is why I have always needed to do both, I guess.

I have been very lucky to have worked with the filmmakers I did work with in the '70s and the '80s, but along the way there were a lot of scripts that didn't get on, like *Dune,* with Ridley Scott. I introduced a few things into the script that weren't in the book and that Frank Herbert really didn't like—I think that is why it didn't get on. Writing an adaptation can be very difficult. Since then I prefer to adapt books—not always, but for the most part—that aren't so well known, or aren't even that good, because then you feel a lot freer.

The only adaptation that I have ever done which is pretty close to the book is *Voyager,*[2] a film I did in Germany with Volcker Schlondorff. Volcker is tremendously well read and very aware of the pitfalls of adaptation, I think a lot of what was good about that script came about because of the close collaboration with Volcker.

Anyway, as L.A. became more and more problematic, I chose more of an independent route, which was difficult. I began to work much more in Europe, with people like Volcker and Alex Cox, [Michelangelo] Antonioni and [Bernardo] Bertolucci and Jacques Dorfmann, a French director. I was much more comfortable working in that way even though there were lean times. The few times that I went back to L.A., when I was really broke and had to take a job for the money—they were always a disaster and I usually regretted it.

ALEX COX AND *WALKER*

I had a wonderful time working with Alex Cox on *Walker.* He left me to my own ends on the script, as well as infusing the process with a rare degree of equality, which made it even more important to find out what he wanted. It was a real collaboration in the sense that we were constantly excited by each other's ideas. We did a couple of other scripts together afterwards which we never got produced, but we had a fun and crazy time making *Walker.*

I usually start with a rough outline which I give myself total permission to change as I go along. I like to write a really quick first draft and set it aside and go ponder, before heading into another draft. I don't show the first draft to anyone except for a few friends for a few comments and to get a general sense of how it plays . . . , but each script and each film is different.

We made *Walker* for very little money in Nicaragua so the studio left us alone during the shooting. Once we were in Nicaragua, we were in our own world. The Sandanista government was supportive. They were fairly open and generous, with an innocence about how a film got made. But it was a very good experience. Anyone who was working on the film was very impassioned, and we all went a little crazy in the good sense of the word.

Universal was very frightened by the film, partly because it was shot in Nicaragua at a time when that country wasn't very popular with the Reagan administration. They put it on the shelf for a long time. Partly they didn't understand the deliberate use of anachronisms to suggest the timelessness of imperialism. Not very many critics did either. Alex says that concept was mine, but I say it was his idea. I didn't really want to do that, but now, today, when I watch the re-release from Criterion, it works so much better than it did then. I was nervous because once you break a certain taboo you are asking for critical rejection, which certainly happened. That concept really makes sense, but it also really alienated a lot of people . . . certainly the more conservative element of the audience.

Traditional liberals were very uneasy about the whole film also. *Walker* had a little too much anarchy and it imposed a certain conceptual view and it really risked a lot. The risk taking is to Alex's credit. He is a ferocious filmmaker. The score itself, by Joe Strummer, is probably one of the best film scores I have ever been involved with, apart from the Dylan score for *Pat Garrett.*

ANTONIONI AND "TWO TELEGRAMS"

My relationship with Antonioni was amazing. He first asked me to do a script based on a short piece he wrote called "Two Telegrams." I worked with him in Rome. I was in love with Antonioni's work and felt that it was a great privilege to be around him and to witness and observe him. But then halfway through the process, in 1985, he had a massive stroke that made it very difficult to work, because he couldn't speak or walk; but he was still tremendously determined to get the film made. We spent time in L.A. because it was supposed to be shot there, and we had endless meetings with actors and stuff; and the title kept changing. But it was sort of like "The Emperor's New Clothes": no one could say no to the maestro. While at the same time there was a growing sense that he could never get bonded and there had to be another director as a backup—I think it was going to be Atom Egoyan.

At some point it became clear that we were just working to keep him going. The writing of the script was in a sense meant to keep him alive. I was really happy to continue working with him, though, because he was an extraordinary person, difficult at times, but really great and a real artist. I spent many years working on and off on "Two Telegrams."

CARROLL BALLARD AND *WIND*

Wind was a frustrating film, because Carroll Ballard and I went to Australia and I was writing it just before principal photography. I tried to inhabit the whole process of yacht races as much as I could. Carroll is a consummate cinematographer with a rare and fluid visual appreciation of film, but he is very insecure about narrative and character and he had a lot of problems dealing with the script and actors. He is intensely uncomfortable and insecure with language, which made writing the script difficult and frustrating. To the end, he was always reaching out for other writers, and enlisting changes, many of which didn't work. I stayed on the production as long as I could and then I left because I had given it all I could give.

Antonioni is also a total visualist, who seeks to explore the script through how an image presents itself to him and how it fits with his obsession with certain kinds of images. But Antonioni had an incredible appreciation for language as long as it serves the visual process. That was something I could relate to. He was the master of his domain, and there was never any confusion about what was right for him, yet one was always in the conversation. There was actually better communication with Antonioni than with Carroll.

BERNARDO BERTOLUCCI AND *LITTLE BUDDHA*

Bernardo is a wonderful director, who has done some great work, but I think he was intimidated by the subject at the heart of *Little Buddha*, a little bit afraid of it, and ultimately he didn't understand the essence of the Buddha's spiritual journey. He hid behind a magic children's tale. Having lived and studied in India and Nepal, I think I knew too much about the subject to be objective and to feel comfortable with that approach. While it was an interesting project, it was frustrating because I felt it could have been a tougher and much more rigorous film, rather than a film that was hiding behind Keanu Reeves. I don't know how to say this in a gentle way because I respect Bertolucci a lot, but I just felt he took too reductive an approach to the subject and made too much of a Hollywood film.

Mark Peploe, his brother-in-law, came in at the end to finish the writing. It was a complicated time for me because my stepson had just been killed in a car crash and I was a more than a little bit out of it. *Little Buddha* was not a good experience because I had the rug pulled out from underneath me. I wasn't prepared for Peploe's involvement. But I am still glad to have worked for Bernardo, and I shifted to a different state of mind. That is when I wrote my book *Hard Travel to Sacred Places*, about my stepson's death, and about traveling to Southeast Asia—Cambodia, Burma, and Thailand—with my wife, Lynn Davis.

I've always tried to sign on to a project with a director that I respected, who offered a sense of sharing common ground. It's a director's medium and after thirty or so years of writing scripts I find it increasingly difficult if not impossible to sublimate myself to someone else's vision unless I respect him, particularly if there's no sense of collaboration. Each film is different, and each has its own dilemmas and solutions, but the writer is in a sublimated position—especially sublimated to the director's authority—and I have to respect the director. It's is a complicated process, and for me, the process is as much about my own explorations and finding out what I really think, rather than about what somebody else thinks. Sometimes you get lucky and you can meet in the middle, where there is genuine give and take. You are both helping the other to find out about themselves.

RETURN TO PROSE

A novel offers total creative freedom and autonomy, compared to the restrictions and frustrations of mining the celluloid trail. Film, for a writer, is often a two-dimensional medium limited to a ninety- or hundred-minute time frame. The novel, on the other hand, is open ended, and involves four or more dimensions as well as a chance to explore hidden layers and internal complexities.

I always have felt the need to express myself in a more interior way. I always intended to move back and forth between film and books, with those two careers kind of coexisting. They did for a while, and particularly in the '70s you could be much freer with scripts and you could be more autonomous in your film work. When you were dealing with Hellman, Peckinpah, or Hal Ashby, it was freer; there was more equality in the collaboration, and more enjoyment in writing the scripts. Then it became a longer and longer process, and more difficult because you had more people to relate to and more commercial elements, so the time between scripts and books became longer.

With *The Drop Edge of Yonder* I found I was able to include much of what I learned from writing scripts, particularly as that novel originated in several old scripts.

One was a script I had written in the '70s about a mountain man: "Zebulon," which several directors, including Peckinpah, Ashby, Roger Spottiswode, Alex Cox, and others, were enthusiastic about and tried to get funded. But due to Peckinpah's and then Ashby's death, as well as the fashions of the L.A. film business, the script drifted for years, almost but never quite being realized. I also wrote a script for Mike Medavoy about the Gold Rush, which never got on. These and other similar projects involved enormous research, which I continued on my own, as I had become somewhat obsessed with the origins and eccentricities of the American frontier in all its themes of exploration, greed, violence, freedom, and so on.

All the research was on my palette, so to speak, and I was so frustrated about the fate of these various scripts that after *Little Buddha* I sat down and wrote this novel that had nothing to do with any of these scripts, really, except they were something of a catalyst, and the novel represents a kind of fusion of screenwriting and a prose approach. *The Drop Edge of Yonder* is, at least on the surface, an old-fashioned yarn, like an eighteenth-century novel about the nineteenth century, with twenty-first-century chords and complexities. Because the origins came from a few old scripts, the rhythm of the book is very cinematic; many of the paragraphs that open chapters are like silent master shots, exploring and establishing space and movement, then continuing with dialogue, action, and character exploration—which, in turn, finally dissolves into the next chapter and another master shot. And so on. There are still elements of Samuel Beckett's influence—the internal through-line is very circular, rather than linear, and there are residues of my early novels—but because of the cinematic style people have found *The Drop Edge of Yonder* more accessible and certainly less solipsistic and more entertaining. I wasn't trying to do that; that is just how it evolved.

THE CORPORATIZATION OF FILM

Films cost way too much money and have to play across the board to a whole swathe of audiences. They have become more and more simplistic and dumbed-down. The writing is dumbed-down. Oddly, the best writing these days tends to be on TV, where language seems to be more honored.

I worked with Sidney Lumet on this TV series that Alan Arkin was in [*100 Centre Street*], and it was so much more enjoyable. Lumet is one of a kind, but he values language and was totally professional without any thought about the level of the audience he was reaching for. I was totally surprised by the experience, and given the right situation I would work in television again. A miniseries or something.

I have been working a little bit off and on with Arkin on a script and I love working with him because he is so much fun and creative. He has written and directed himself. He's fabulous. We do that because we have fun doing it; I don't know what will happen with it.

There have been a few film scripts since *Little Buddha*. There was a film called *Shadow of the Wolf*, which took place in the Arctic, which I was always interested in, But it was not a good film. The director was very scared of the terrain. It wasn't a great experience. I have worked on some Canadian films because along the way I landed immigrant status in Canada; most recently I worked with Bille August on a script that is supposed to be shot this fall, but we'll see. I have tried to ease myself gradually out of the grid of Hollywood. I suppose I'm a marginal character where Hollywood is concerned.

That one word *industry* says it all. When you have this plan about what the process should be and how you should think about it, you are three-fourths dead before you even start. There's a certain amount of solitude that is involved with writing and discovery, and when you try to map it out conceptually as to what the form is—beginning, middle, and end, and this and that—to me, that's a disaster. Film schools have been a disaster for writing. And then you go into some producer's room, and there are four or five people there, and three or four of them are sales or marketing and development people, and you have to pitch what you want to do, and then they give you your notes.

By the time you are finished with all that you no longer want to write the script. You are sort of dead in the water. Then the writing of the script becomes really heavy lifting, not a generous or nourishing process. One of the great things about working with Monte Hellman so early in my career is that all he said to me was, "I want to read something from you that I haven't read before." That was great; then I could surprise myself. When you try to eliminate that element of surprise or discovery, then why do it?

Every time I think of sitting down and writing a screenplay in recent years, I try to wait until the thought passes *[laughs]*. "Let's get that cloud out of the sky."

At this stage of life, it becomes a question of how free you can be. You have to feel a certain intensity about things. You just don't want to waste time. Unless you are protected, unless you feel comfortable with people, for me it's not worth doing. Who knows what will fly up and hit your windshield?

June 2008

RUDY WURLITZER (1938–)

1965	*Birth of the Flag I* and *II* (short subjects). Director.
1971	*Glen and Randa* (Jim McBride). Co-script.
	Two-Lane Blacktop (Monte Hellman). Co-Script.
1973	*Pat Garrett and Billy the Kid* (Sam Peckinpah). Script, actor.
1975	*Keep Busy* (Robert Frank). Script, actor.
1977	*Coming Home* (Hal Ashby). Uncredited contribution.
1981	*Energy and How to Get It* (Robert Frank). Script.
1986	*America* (Robert Downey, Sr.). Actor.
1987	*Walker* (Alex Cox). Script.
	Candy Mountain (Robert Frank, Rudy Wurlitzer). Co-director, script.
	Malone (Harley Cokeliss). Uncredited contribution.
1991	*Voyager / Homo Faber* (Volker Schlondorff). Script.
1992	*Little Buddha* (Bernardo Bertolucci). Co-script.
	Wind (Carroll Ballard). Co-script.
	Shadow of the Wolf (Jacques Dorfmann / Pierre Magny). Co-script.

Television credits include the documentary *The Spirit of Tibet* (1995); one episode of the HBO series *Strangers* (1996); and episodes of *100 Centre Street* (2001–2), produced by Sidney Lumet for A&E.

Novels include *Nog; Flats; Quake; Slow Fade;* and *The Drop Edge of Yonder.* Other books include the memoir *Hard Travel to Sacred Places,* and the published screenplays of *Two-Lane Blacktop* and *Walker.*[3]

NOTES

1 "Two Telegrams" is a short story or sketch that is included in the collection *That Bowling Alley on the Tiber: Tales of a Director,* by Michelangelo Antonioni (1989).

2 *Voyager* is based on *Homo Faber: A Report,* a 1957 novel by the highly regarded Swiss architect, playwright, and author Max Frisch.

3 Wurlitzer's novels and screenplays are the focus of David Seed's critical monograph *Rudolph Wurlitzer: American Novelist and Screenwriter* (1992). A near exhaustive listing of his works, interviews, and reviews can be found on the writer's own Web site, www.rudywurlitzer.com.

ABOUT THE CONTRIBUTORS

A writer-director from Copenhagen, Denmark, **MIKAEL COLVILLE-ANDERSEN** embarked in 1999 on a journey to meet the six greatest living screenwriters in Europe and shoot a documentary. Jean-Claude Carrière was one of them, if not the greatest of the lot. Colville-Andersen has been involved in film and television for over twenty years, and, after graduating from the National Film School of Denmark, he turned his focus to the screenwriting craft and the inspiration gained from his meetings with the masters.

NICK DAWSON writes a weekly interview column, *The Director Interviews,* for *Filmmaker Magazine,* and is an editor at FilmInFocus.com. Originally from the United Kingdom, he has written for *Empire, Uncut,* the *London Times* and the *Scotsman,* and now lives in Brooklyn, New York. His biography of Hal Ashby, *Being Hal Ashby,* was published by the University of Kentucky Press in 2009.

F-STOP FITZGERALD's Web site is www.f-stopfitzgerald.com.

The work of freelance writer **WILLIAM HAM** has appeared in *Lollipop, McSweeney's Internet Concern, Ben Is Dead,* and the *Cambridge Book Review,* among others. Ham is also the cofounder of *The High Hat,* a sporadically published Web site dealing with popular culture (www.thehighhat.com); a contributor to the book *Lost in the Grooves: Scram's Capricious Guide to the Music You Missed;* and the host of *Wow and Flutter,* a biweekly music-comedy show on KMUN-FM, Astoria Oregon. He lives in Ilwaco, Washington, "if you call that living," he says.

LEE HILL interviewed Terry Southern for *Backstory 3*. He is the author of *A Grand Guy,* a biography of Southern, and a BFI Modern Classic on *Easy Rider.* Currently based in London, England, he works as a writer and communications consultant. He has contributed to *Senses of Cinema, Vertigo,*

Scenario, the Canadian Broadcasting Corporation, the *Guardian, Cinemascope,* and other outlets.

VINCENT LOBRUTTO is an instructor of editing, production design, and cinema studies for the Department of Film, Video, and Animation at the School of Visual Arts in New York, where he is a thesis advisor and member of the Thesis Committee. He is the author of *Selected Takes: Film Editors on Editing; By Design: Interviews with Film Production Designers; Sound-on-Film: Interviews with Creators of Film Sound; Stanley Kubrick: A Biography; Principal Photography: Interviews with Feature Film Cinematographers; The Filmmaker's Guide to Production Design; The Encyclopedia of American Independent Filmmaking; Becoming Film Literate: The Art and Craft of Motion Pictures; Martin Scorsese: A Biography;* and *The Art of Motion Picture Editing.* A special member of American Cinema Editors (ACE), LoBrutto is the editor of *CinemaEditor* magazine and a contributor to *American Cinematographer, Film Quarterly,* and *Films in Review.*

Himself a screenwriter, **TOM MATTHEWS** wrote the 1997 film *Mad City,* starring Dustin Hoffman and John Travolta, which was directed by Costas-Gavras. He has written scripts for Universal Pictures, Warner Brothers, New Line Cinema, Twentieth Century Fox, and Walt Disney Pictures. His acclaimed satirical novel, *Like We Care,* was published in 2004 by Bancroft Press. His freelance articles have appeared in the *Milwaukee Journal Sentinel, Milwaukee Magazine, Creative Screenwriting,* and *Classic Drummer.* For six years he was the managing editor of *Boxoffice Magazine* in Hollywood.

The editor of the Backstory series, author **PATRICK McGILLIGAN** has written numerous books about film, including the *New York Times* Notable Books *George Cukor: A Double Life* and *Fritz Lang: The Nature of the Beast;* the Edgar-nominated *Alfred Hitchcock: A Life in Darkness and Light;* and, most recently, *Oscar Micheaux: The Great and Only,* which was cited by the New York Public Library as among the "25 Books to Remember" from 2007. With Paul Buhle he also edited the definitive oral history *Tender Comrades, A Backstory of the Blacklist.* McGilligan lives in Milwaukee, Wisconsin.

GAVIN SMITH is editor of *Film Comment.*

GENERAL INDEX

INDEX OF FILMS, PLAYS, AND BOOKS

Text: 10/13 Aldus
Display: Bell Gothic
Compositor: International Typesetting and Composition
Indexer: Roberta Engleman
Printer: Maple-Vail Book Manufacturing Group